VARNEY'S MIDWIFERY

STUDY QUESTION
BOOK

JENIFER O. FAHEY, CNM, MSN, MPH

Clinical Instructor, University of Maryland Medical School

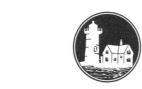

JONES AND BARTLETT PUBLISHERS
Sudbury, Massachusetts
BOSTON   TORONTO   LONDON   SINGAPORE

World Headquarters

Jones and Bartlett Publishers
40 Tall Pine Drive
Sudbury, MA 01776
978-443-5000
info@jbpub.com
www.jbpub.com

Jones and Bartlett Publishers
Canada
2406 Nikanna Road
Mississauga, ON L5C 2W6
CANADA

Jones and Bartlett Publishers
International
Barb House, Barb Mews
London W6 7PA
UK

Copyright © 2002 by Jones and Bartlett Publishers, Inc.

All rights reserved. No part of the material protected by this copyright may be reproduced or utilized in any form, electronic or mechanical, including photocopying, recording, or by any information storage and retrieval system, without written permission from the copyright owner.

Library of Congress Cataloging-in-Publication Data

Fahey, Jenifer.
    Varney's midwifery study question book / by Jenifer Fahey.
        p. cm.
      ISBN 0-7637-1641-3 (pbk.)
        1. Midwives.   2. Midwifery--Examinations--Study guides.   3.
    Midwives--Examinations--Study guides.   I. Varney, Helen. Varney's midwifery.   II. Title.

    RG950.F34 2001
    618.2'0076--dc21   2001038231

Production Credits
Acquisitions Editor: Penny Glynn
Associate Editor: Thomas Prindle
Marketing Manager: Taryn Wahlquist
Production Editor: Jon Workman
Manufacturing Buyer: Amy Duddridge
Text Design: Anne Spencer
Cover Design: Kristin Ohlin
Editorial Production Service: Trillium Management
Typesetting: Northeast Compositors
Printing and Binding: Courier Companies, Inc.
Cover Printing: Courier Companies, Inc.

Printed In the United States of America
05 04 03 02 01   10 9 8 7 6 5 4 3 2 1

For my midwifery classmates with whom I studied (without a midwifery study guide) and who helped teach me the things about being a midwife that one cannot learn from books—compassion, patience, perseverance, and, most important, loyalty.

ACKNOWLEDGEMENTS

Needless to say, this book would not have been possible without Helen Varney Burst whose text, *Varney's Midwifery*, was not only a nearly constant companion through my midwifery education, but also provided the springboard for this project. Helen's role in this endeavor, however, goes far deeper than her provision of the textbook and of much "technical" advice and assistance. She speaks of the "Guardian Angels" in her third edition; well, Helen is the guardian angel of the Yale Midwifery Class of 2000. Her love for the profession and for her students is downright contagious and I am most fortunate to count myself among those she has mentored.

Thanks go as well to Carolyn Gegor and Jan Kriebs for taking a chance on me three times and for all their hard work in revising the manuscript for this book. I am honored to be able to work with them on this book and as a member of their team at the University of Maryland.

My classmates, to whom I have dedicated this book, deserve many thanks for serving as a constant source of advice, inspiration, and encouragement. They have always believed in me and helped give wings to a series of projects, including this one.

I am grateful for my publishing team at Jones and Bartlett for their vote of confidence and for their hard work in bringing this book to production. Special thanks to Christine Tridente, my editor, who kept me on task with a series of gentle and encouraging e-mails and who helped kick me into high-gear to get this book completed with a not-so-gentle e-mail!

Congratulations and thanks to Midshipman Jason Chen for the illustrations that accompany some of the questions in this book—I don't think the US Naval Academy has ever had a student so well versed in midwifery!

Thanks to the women and babies for whom I have been fortunate enough to provide care—they have taught me volumes about myself as a person and as a midwife.

Finally, a special thank you to my wonderful and loving husband, Sean, for being infinitely patient and for creating a space (in time and place) where I could work on the book without distractions. This has been especially important in the last couple of months during which I have started working at the University of Maryland and since our most important project, our first child (now in gestation), has needed more of my time and energy.

TABLE OF CONTENTS

INTRODUCTION

As several of my classmates and I gathered to study one evening, I noticed that strewn on my dining room table and balanced over the backs of chairs were a dozen or so study guides. The group had done a thorough job of scouring the local bookstores and the Internet in search of study guides that would help us in the endeavor of successfully sitting for the ACC examination, a prerequisite for certification within our chosen profession. All the books we found, including those that we purchased, were written either to prepare medical students for their board examination, adult nurse practitioners for their professional exam, or nursing students for the national nursing licensing exam, the NCLEX. None of these study guides, therefore, addressed the topics particular to the practice of midwifery and were, thus, of limited usefulness. Undoubtedly, our small study group was neither the first nor the last congregation of midwifery students to note with much frustration the dearth, if not complete absence, of study guides written for us.

As I considered the possibility of addressing this vacuum in the educational materials available to midwifery students, it made most sense to turn to *Varney's Midwifery*—a text written with the expressed goal of addressing the learning needs of individuals preparing to practice midwifery. Helen Varney Burst, in the preface to the first edition of her textbook, describes the frustration faced by those "trying to piece together what the practice of nurse-midwifery is from a conglomeration of American nursing and medical literature and English midwifery texts." To address this frustration, she wrote the first American midwifery textbook. It is in this spirit of creating our own body of didactic literature that *Varney's Study Question Book* was conceived and that I now present it both to students currently undertaking their formal midwifery education and to all students of midwifery.

HOW TO USE THIS STUDY QUESTION BOOK

While a concerted effort was made to write this book to assist students in their preparation for the American College of Nurse-Midwives Certification Council (ACC) exam, that is neither the main nor the sole purpose of this book. This book is intended to serve primarily as a companion learning tool to the third edition of *Varney's Midwifery*. The study outlines were created to help guide and focus your studying. The practice questions are also intended to help your study efforts and to provide valuable practice in taking multiple-choice tests. Before specifically addressing how to best use this book for exam preparation, however, I would like to address some general issues regarding the multiple-choice exam format.

With increasing frequency, the exams administered to midwifery students within their educational programs and to certified nurse-midwives and certified midwives trying to earn continuing education credits (CEC's) are of a multiple-choice format. Successfully completing such exams requires not only knowledge and understanding of the material being tested, but also a familiarity and confidence with multiple-choice questions. An important component of preparing for a multiple-choice exam, therefore, is to practice reading and answering multiple-choice questions. This may make intuitive sense, but nonetheless, many students prepare for multiple-choice exams without practicing these types of questions. This book, more than providing outlines to guide and focus your study, was written to give you this necessary practice in reading and answering multiple-choice questions that were specifically designed to test material relevant to midwifery.

Multiple-choice questions (MCQ's) consist of two basic parts: (a) the "stem," which identifies the question or problem and (b) the response alternatives. Within the response alternatives presented in this book and in the ACC exam, there is one correct answer and two to three incorrect alternatives, known as "distractors."

While multiple-choice questions may have definite drawbacks, they also possess characteristics that make them especially attractive and useful for exams that are administered to a large and varied group of students or that are meant to test students on a broad range of topics and extensive amount of information. These benefits include the following:

- MCQ's are easily scored, which allows for quick turn-around time on test results.

- The scoring of multiple-choice exams can be both accurate and objective, two standards that are difficult to achieve with other exam formats.

- MCQ's can be designed to test a student at different cognitive levels.

- MCQ's allow for testing on a broad scope of topics.

- It is easy to gather statistics on multiple-choice questions, and these statistics can be used to rank questions with respect to their difficulty and their ability to discriminate between students of different competency levels.

Multiple-choice exams will *not* test for all you know. The sooner you can accept this fact, the sooner you can focus on improving your performance on these tests. It is impossible for any exam, let alone one using only multiple-choice questions, to assess your entire knowledge base or your mastery of clinical skills—this is why your faculty members and preceptors have assessed your skills in the clinical setting, why you are asked to present case studies, and why you will also take exams that will use short-answers or essay questions.

Do not prepare for your exams through gaming strategy. Contrary to student lore, option "C" is not really statistically more likely to be the correct answer. Many of the exams that you will take—especially the ACC exam—are written by experts both in the field of midwifery and in the field of test design. You can rest assured that they have taken all possible measures to avoid multiple-choice question pitfalls, such as accidentally divulging the answer through grammatical clues in the question stems.

This being said, there are some steps you can take to become a better multiple-choice exam taker. The following are some of the main steps to success in taking multiple-choice exams:

- Read the question stem thoroughly, and more than once if necessary. Make sure that you understand what the question is asking. Make note of or underline words such as "most," "least," "true," "false," "not," and so on. Watch for negative or positive phrasing, or qualifying words like "always" or "never," which can drastically change the meaning of a statement.

- Try to answer the question on your own. In other words, when you read the stem, if possible, answer the question in your mind before looking at the answer choices. You will then be able to look at the answer choices to find which one best matches your own answer. As you read through the possible responses, mark off the ones you know are wrong. If none of the answer options seems close, reread the question. If you still cannot answer the item, move on to the next item. Before moving on, however, clearly mark those questions that you need to come back to later. Remember that it is possible that something, such as another question, may trigger your memory and make it easier to answer the questions you skipped earlier.

- If the "distractors" are written well, there will often be more than one answer choice that seems correct. Your task is to choose the *best* or *most appropriate* answer. Remember that the right answer is *not* always the same thing as what you see done most often in clinical practice. There should always be sound theoretical/statistical basis for your response.

- Time yourself. It is important not to rush through questions, but it is also important not to spend more time than necessary on items to which you do not know the answer. One of the advantages of multiple-choice exams is that more often than not the items are equally weighted. In other words, the questions that you *do* know the answer to are worth as much the one you don't know.

- Practice! Practice! Practice! Which brings us to the next section. . .

Varney's Study Question Book was written as a companion book to the third edition of *Varney's Midwifery*. Questions are drawn directly from the body of the text, and the answer keys include the page numbers of the mother book from which the question and the correct answer were drawn. In several instances, the information contained in *Varney's Pocket Midwife* (also a companion book to the third edition of *Varney's Midwifery*) is either more up-to-date or is presented in a manner that facilitates question formulation. In these instances, the page numbers provided in the answer keys include the initials "PM" to denote that the question and answer were drawn from the *Pocket Midwife* rather than from the "mother book."

The study question book is divided in sections that roughly mirror the sections in *Varney's Midwifery*. There is not, however, a chapter-to-chapter correlation. For example, each of the methods of contraception has an individual chapter devoted to it in the mother book. In this book they are all combined into one chapter. Similarly, most of the clinical skills chapters have been merged into other chapters where the information fits best. Questions on bimanual compression, for example, are included in the section on abnormalities of third and fourth stages of labor.

The questions in the book were designed to test different levels of the midwifery management process/framework. Some questions will ask you to identify a problem or make a diagnosis while others will ask you to form a management plan. In other words, some questions will test your knowledge while others will test your clinical judgment and clinical decision-making skills.

I have included study outlines at the beginning of each section and I have made every attempt to make them as comprehensive as possible, but they are by no means an exhaustive list of the material you have learned or for which you are responsible. You can use these outlines to guide and/or focus your study. The study outlines include material that is not in the mother book but that should be considered "fair game" for the ACC examination. While general well-woman/gynecologic care is included, there is not a full primary care section. The next edition of *Varney's Midwifery* and, therefore, the next edition of this book, will include a primary care section that addresses such issues as asthma, diabetes, hypertension, etc. These changes, like changes in the ACC exam, are made to reflect the expanding role of midwifery in the United States.

At the end of the book you will find two practice tests with questions drawn from all the sections in the book. These practice tests are a little less than approximately half the length of the ACC examination and, like the ACC exam, present questions in random order rather than grouped according to topic areas. Also like the ACC exam, the practice tests are composed of questions that test both knowledge and clinical judgment. Approximately two-thirds of the questions will test on normal phenomena while one-third will be devoted to deviations from normal. I suggest that you save these practice tests for a time that you can sit down and take them all at once and time yourself. You should give yourself 90 minutes to complete each exam.

In addition to using this book to practice reading and answering multiple choice questions, you can use the questions, the outlines, and the practice test to pinpoint your areas of weakness. This will allow you to focus and prioritize your studying efforts. Some students have a weakness related to test-taking skills (not pacing themselves or missing key words in the stems), others may have gaps in their knowledge of specific content areas, and still others may have a weakness in answering questions that test a particular level of the management framework (data base vs. management plan).

Please note that while it is my intent that this book will help you to prepare for midwifery exams, including the ACC exam, it is not meant to be used as your sole study tool. Furthermore, any information included here regarding the ACC exam should not be used in lieu of the information included in the publication "Information For Candidates of The National Certification Examination in Nurse-Midwifery and Midwifery"—a must-read for all individuals preparing for the ACC examination.

I truly hope that you find this study question book enjoyable and useful. Most importantly, I hope that this book will alleviate at least some of the frustration of not having a study guide of "our own."

PART I: MIDWIFERY

Chapter 1: History of Midwifery and Professional Issues

Chapter 1 Outline
History of Midwifery and Professional Issues

I.   Definitions of Midwifery

II. Paths to Midwifery

   A. Nursing and midwifery

   B. Lay midwives, direct-entry midwives, and nurse-midwives
   1. Definitions
   2. Scope of practice
   3. Relationships
   4. National Midwifery/Professional organizations
      a. ACNM
      b. MANA
      c. NARM
      d. MEAC

III. History of Midwifery

   A. Historical roots of midwifery

   B. Midwifery in the United States

   C. Historical trends in midwifery practice, education, and credentialing

IV. International Midwifery

   A. WHO definition of midwifery

   B. The International Confederation of Midwives

   C. The Safe Motherhood Initiative

V.   Midwifery and Medicine

   A. Joint Statement of Practice Relationships Between Obstetricians/Gynecologists and Certified-Nurse Midwives

   B. Relationships
   1. Consultation
   2. Collaboration
   3. Referral

VI. The American College of Nurse-Midwives (ACNM)

   A. Structure and function

   B. The ACNM Documents

   C. The ACNM Foundation

   D. The ACNM's Certification Council (ACC)

VII. Professional Regulation
   A. Accreditation
   B. Credentialing
   C. Licensing
   D. Certification
   E. Prescriptive authority
   F. Hospital privileges
   G. Federal Trade Commission

VIII. Professional Codes/Code of Ethics/Ethics in Midwifery Practice

IX. Legal Issues
   A. Informed consent
   B. Practice standards
   C. Scope of practice
   D. Malpractice
   E. Malpractice insurance
   F. Liability
   G. Risk management

X. The Midwifery Management Process

Chapter 1 Questions
History of Midwifery and Professional Issues

■ **DATA FOR ITEM 1**

"The process whereby a certified nurse-midwife and physician jointly manage the care of a woman or newborn who has become medically, gynecologically, or obstetrically complicated."

1. Which of the following terms is defined above?
  a. Consultation
  b. Collaboration
  c. Referral
  d. Transfer

2. In which of the following ways does the scope of nurse-midwifery practice as defined by the American College of Nurse-Midwives (ACNM) differ from the scope of midwifery practice outlined in the international definition of midwifery accepted by the International Confederation of Midwives and the World Health Organization?
  a. In the birth settings in which midwifery-managed birth can take place
  b. In the type of medical conditions that can be independently managed
  c. In the inclusion of primary health care of women and newborns
  d. In the inclusion of family planning and health education

3. Which of the following is the significant result of the Children's Bureau's first activities?
  a. The opening of the first maternity center in New York City
  b. Increasing the access of midwives to hospitals
  c. Establishing the importance of prenatal care to reducing infant mortality
  d. Founding the Frontier Nursing Service

4. Which of the following women was associated with the founding and successes of the Frontier Nursing Service?
  a. Florence Wald
  b. Mary Breckinridge
  c. Hazel Corbin
  d. Hattie Hemschemeyer

5. Before 1900, what percentage of births took place in the hospital?
  a. 5%
  b. 10%
  c. 20%
  d. 30%

6. When did nurse-midwives gain professional access to hospitals?
  a. 1920s
  b. 1940s
  c. 1950s
  d. 1960s

7. Which of the following statements regarding credentialing of non-nurse midwives is TRUE?
  a. The ACNM's Division of Accreditation (DOA) has developed criteria for midwifery education programs for non-midwives but the ACNM's Certification Council (ACC) will neither test nor certify non-nurse midwives.
  b. There is an agency unrelated to the ACNM that is responsible for the accreditation of midwifery education programs for non-midwives and that administers testing and provides certification for non-nurse midwives.

c. The ACNM's Division of Accreditation (DOA) has developed criteria for midwifery education programs for non-midwives and the ACNM Certification Council (ACC) tests and certifies non-nurse midwives.

d. A non-nurse midwife must complete training as a nurse within an ACNM DOA-accredited program before he or she can sit for the ACC examination and receive ACC certification.

8. Which of the following statements describes a direct-entry midwifery program?

    a. An apprenticeship program to train non-nurse midwives

    b. A program that only accepts students who are already Registered Nurses

    c. A program that provides a midwifery education for individuals who are not, and do not desire to become, Registered Nurses

    d. A program for non-nurses that combines nursing and midwifery education for individuals who are not, but do desire to become, Registered Nurses

9. In what year was the American College of Nurse-Midwives (ACNM) incorporated?

    a. 1954

    b. 1955

    c. 1956

    d. 1969

10. Which of the following steps is NOT included in the ACNM Guidelines for the Incorporation of New Procedures into Nurse-Midwifery Practice?

    a. Identify the need for the procedure

    b. Evaluate the procedure as a nurse-midwifery function

    c. Evaluate the financial costs and potential profitability of the procedure

    d. Develop a process for educating nurse-midwives to perform the procedure

DATA FOR ITEM 11

A certified nurse-midwife has just started clinical practice at the same place where you work. She asks you about the possibility of adding surgical abortion to the services provided at your site.

11. Which of the following statements would be an accurate response?

    a. Nurse-midwives may provide abortion counseling, information on abortion, and nursing care to women having an abortion, but federal law prohibits them from performing abortion procedures.

    b. There exists an ACNM clinical practice statement that prohibits nurse-midwives from performing abortions.

    c. There exists an ACNM document on reproductive choices that lists abortion as a procedure that midwives are able to provide to their clients.

    d. The American College of Obstetricians and Gynecologists (ACOG) has proposed that "mid-level" practitioners such as nurse-midwives perform abortions to increase the availability of safe abortion services.

12. Which of the following statements BEST describes the midwife's main role in the process of differential diagnosis?

    a. Determining the proper diagnosis through history, physical exam, and laboratory studies and then independently managing, collaborating on, or referring the woman's medical care as necessary

    b. Differentiating normal processes from abnormal processes and then independently managing, collaborating on, or referring the woman's medical care as necessary

    c. Formulating a list of possible diagnoses and then consulting with a physician to determine the best course of action

    d. Initiating the process of confirming or ruling out possible diagnoses and then consulting with a physician to make a final diagnosis and determine a course of action

Chapter 1 Answer Key
History of Midwifery and Professional Issues

1. *b* p. 24

2. *c* p. 3, 23

3. *c* p. 6

4. *b* p. 7–8

5. *a* p. 535

6. *c* p. 535

7. *c* p. 15

8. *c* p. 16

9. *b* p. 17

10. *c* p. 349–350 PM

11. *d* p. 253

12. *b* p. 28

PART II: PRIMARY CARE

Chapter 2: Gynecologic/Primary Care of Women

Chapter 3: Methods of Contraception

Chapter 4: Care of the Perimenopausal/ Postmenopausal Woman

Chapter 5: Care of the HIV-Infected Woman and Other Special Primary Care Situations

Chapter 2 Outline
Gynecologic/Primary Care of Women

I.   **Preventive Health Screening Recommendations**

     A. Physical Examination

     B. Immunizations

     C. Breast Examination (Self exam/Professional exam)

     D. Mammography

     E. Pelvic Examination

     F. Pap Smears

     G. Rectal Examination/Occult Stool Blood

     H. Colonoscopy/Proctosigmoidoscopy

     I. Skin Examination (Self exam/Professional exam)

II.   **Normal Anatomy and Physiology of the Breast**

III.   **Breast Masses**

     A. Predisposing factors for breast cancer

     B. Breast examination technique

     C. Characteristic of malignant vs. benign breast masses

         1. Size

         2. Contour

         3. Consistency

         4. Mobility

         5. Enlargement of axillary/supraclavicular lymph nodes

         6. Nipple discharge

         7. Skin changes/Rashes

     D. Management of abnormal findings on breast examinations

         1. Ultrasound evaluation

         2. Needle aspiration/Cytologic analysis of aspirate

         3. Mammography (Screening vs. diagnostic)

         4. Open/Excisional biopsy

IV.   **Normal Reproductive Tract/Pelvic Anatomy**

     A. Ovaries

     B. Uterus/Fallopian Tubes

     C. Cervix

D. Vagina
    1. Vaginal flora and discharge
    2. Bartholin's and Skene's gland

E. Pelvic bones

F. Pelvic muscles

G. Bladder and Urethra

H. Rectum

V.   Papanicolaou (Pap) Smears

A. Technique

B. Indication(s)/Frequency

C. Predisposing factors for pre-cancerous and cancerous cervical lesions

D. Pap Classification Systems

E. Interpretation and Management of Results
    1. Follow-up/Repeat Pap Smears
    2. Colposcopy
    3. Endocervical curettage (ECC)/Biopsy

F. Treatment of Patients with Pre-Cancerous and Cancerous Cervical Lesions
    1. Cryotherapy
    2. Laser conization
    3. Cold knife conization
    4. Loop electrosurgical excision procedure (LEEP)
    5. Management of abnormal pap smears in pregnancy

VI.   Physiology of the Menstrual Cycle

A. Hormonal regulation of the menstrual cycle
    1. Gonadotropin-releasing hormone (GnRH)
    2. Luteinizing hormone (LH)
    3. Follicle-stimulating hormone (FSH)
    4. Estrogen
    5. Progesterone

B. Phases of the Menstrual Cycle
    1. Follicular phase
    2. Ovulatory phase
    3. Luteal phase
    4. Menstrual phase

C. Characteristics of Normal Menses
    1. Frequency
    2. Duration
    3. Amount

VII. Abnormal Uterine Bleeding

A. Definition
  1. Polymenorrhea
  2. Menorrhagia
  3. Metrorrhagia
  4. Menometrorrhagia
  5. Intermenstrual bleeding
  6. Postcoital bleeding
  7. Oligomenorrhea
  8. Postmenopausal bleeding

B. Etiology
  1. Pregnancy
  2. Systemic disease
  3. Organic disease
  4. Dysfunctional Uterine Bleeding (DUB)
    a. Anovulatory vs. Ovulatory

C. Evaluation/Differential Diagnosis
  1. History/Menstrual History
  2. Physical Exam
    a. Speculum exam to rule out vaginal and/or cervical abnormalities
    b. Bimanual exam
    c. Abdominal exam
  3. Labs
    a. Pregnancy test
    b. CBC (Hemoglobin and Hematocrit)
    c. Coagulation studies
    d. Thyroid function tests
    e. Prolactin levels
    f. Liver panel
    g. Follicle-stimulating hormone (FSH)/Luteinizing hormone (LH) levels
    h. Androgen levels
  4. Endometrial Biopsy
  5. Imaging Studies

D. Treatment
  1. Nonsteroidal anti-inflammatory agents (NSAIDs)
  2. Hormonal therapies
    a. Combination oral contraceptives
    b. Cyclic progestin
    c. Depot-medroxyprogesterone acetate (DMPA)
    d. Danazol
    e. GnRH agonists
    f. Progestin IUD
  3. Surgical therapies

VIII. Amenorrhea

A. Definition

    1. Primary vs. Secondary

B. Etiology

C. Evaluation/Differential Diagnosis

    1. History/Menstrual History/Medication and Drug Usage

    2. Physical Exam

        a. Signs/Symptoms galactorrhea

        b. Signs/Symptoms androgen excess

        c. Signs/Symptoms thyroid dysfunction

    3. Labs

        a. Pregnancy test

        b. Thyroid-stimulating hormone (TSH) levels

        c. Follicle-stimulating hormone (FSH) levels

        d. Androgen levels

    4. Progestin Challenge Test

D. Management and Treatment

IX. Dysmenorrhea

A. Definition

    1. Primary vs. Secondary

B. Evaluation/Differential Diagnosis

    1. Physiologic

    2. Adenomyosis

    3. Endometriosis

    4. Pelvic adhesions

C. Management and Treatment

    1. Comfort/Relief measures

    2. Nonsteroidal anti-inflammatory agents (NSAIDs)

    3. Combination oral contraceptives (bicycling/tricycling)

    4. Depot-medroxyprogesterone acetate (DMPA)

X. Premenstrual Syndrome (PMS)

A. Definition

B. Signs/Symptoms

C. Management/Treatment

XI. Toxic Shock Syndrome (TSS)

A. Definition

B. Etiology

C. Signs/Symptoms

D. Management/Treatment

XII.   Intrauterine Exposure to Diethylstilbestrol (DES)

A. Definition

B. Signs/Symptoms

C. Sequelae of intrauterine exposure to DES

D. Management/Treatment
   1. Pap smears

XIII.   Vulvovaginitis/Gynecologic Infections

   • Bacterial Vaginosis

   • Candida Vaginitis (Candidiasis)

   • Trichomonads Vaginitis

   • Atrophic Vaginitis

   • Bartholinitis

Know the following about each of the above conditions:

A. Causative Agent(s)

B. Predisposing Factors

C. Diagnosis
   1. History
   2. Physical Exam
      a. Lesions, erythema, swelling, tenderness of vagina and cervix
      b. Discharge: color, amount, texture, distribution, and odor
   3. Wet Mount
      a. Clue Cells
      b. Buds and Hyphae
      c. Trichomonads
      d. Leukocytes
      e. Erythrocytes
      f. pH of discharge
      g. Amine (Whiff) test

D. Treatment/Relief Measures

XIV.   Sexually Transmitted Infections

   • Herpes Simplex Virus (HSV)

   • Human Papilloma Virus (HPV)/Condylomata Acuminata

   • Molluscum Contagiosum

   • Chancroid

   • Chlamydia

   • Gonorrhea

- Syphilis
- Pelvic Inflammatory Disease

Know the following about each of the above infections:

A. Causative Agent/Predisposing Factors

B. Signs and Symptoms

C. Diagnosis
  1. History
  2. Physical Exam
     a. Lesions on vulva, vagina, cervix, perineal/perianal regions
  3. Cultures/Biopsies/Pap Smear

D. Treatment
  1. CDC Guidelines for Treatment of Sexually Transmitted Diseases
  2. Cryotherapy
  3. Surgical excision

E. Possible Sequelae of Infection

F. Impact on Pregnancy/Childbirth

G. Preventive Measures/Safer Sex Education

XV. Endometriosis

A. Definition

B. Predisposing Factors

C. Signs/Symptoms

D. Diagnosis
  1. Laproscopy

E. Management/Treatment
  1. Relief/Comfort measures
  2. Hormonal/Medical treatment
  3. Surgical treatment

XVI. Pelvic Masses

A. Fibroids/Adenomyosis
  1. Definition
  2. Etiology
  3. Predisposing factors
  4. Signs/Symptoms
  5. Diagnosis
  6. Management/Treatment

B. Ovarian Masses
  1. Etiology
  2. Predisposing factors
  3. Signs/Symptoms

4. Diagnosis

5. Management/Treatment

XVII. Urinary Tract Infections (UTI's)

A. Cystitis/Recurrent Cystitis

    1. Definition

    2. Etiology/Causative organisms

    3. Predisposing factors

    4. Signs/Symptoms

    5. Diagnosis

    6. Management/Treatment

        a. Comfort/Relief measures

        b. Preventive measures

B. Pyelonephritis

    1. Definition

    2. Etiology/Causative organisms

    3. Predisposing factors

    4. Signs/Symptoms

    5. Diagnosis

    6. Management/Treatment

XVIII. Urinary Incontinence

A. Definition/Classification

B. Etiology

C. Predisposing factors

D. Evaluation/Diagnosis

E. Management/Treatment

    1. Kegel's exercises

XIX. Pelvic Relaxation

Cystocele

Urethrocele

Rectocele

Enterocele

Uterine Prolapse

A. Definition/Classification

B. Etiology

C. Predisposing factors

D. Diagnosis

E. Management/Treatment

    1. Kegel's exercises

XX. Infertility

A. Definition

B. Etiology

C. Predisposing factors

D. Diagnosis

E. Management/Treatment

XXI. Pelvic Pain

A. Acute vs. Chronic

B. Evaluation/Differential Diagnosis

(See Table 1 at the end of this section for: "Differential Diagnosis of Pelvic Pain")

C. History (The Seven Characteristics of Pain)
  1. Onset
  2. Location
  3. Character/Type
  4. Duration
  5. Radiation
  6. Associated symptoms
  7. Alleviating/Aggravating factors

D. Physical exam
  1. Vital signs
  2. Abdominal exam
  3. Pelvic exam
  4. Bimanual/Rectovaginal exam

E. Labs/Diagnostic Tests
  1. Pregnancy test
  2. CBC
  3. Urinalysis/Urine culture and sensitivity
  4. Endocervical cultures
  5. Pelvic ultrasound
  6. Radiographic studies
  7. Culdocentesis
  8. Laproscopy

F. Management/Treatment

▪ Table 1: Differential Diagnosis of Pelvic Pain

Pregnancy
   Abortion
   Ectopic pregnancy
Ovary
   Ovarian cysts
   Ruptured ovarian cyst
   Ovarian torsion
   Tuboovarian abscess
   Mittelschmertz
   Ovarian masses/neoplasms
Fallopian Tubes
   Acute salpingitis/Pelvic inflammatory disease (PID)
   Tuboovarian abscess
   Fallopian tube torsion
Uterus
   Fibroids
   Endometriosis
   Infection/Pelvic inflammatory disease (PID)
   Adenomyosis
   Dysmenorrhea
Urinary Tract
   Cystitis
   Pyelonephritis
   Kidney stones
Gastrointestinal
   Appendicitis
   Infectious diarrhea
   Inflammatory bowel disease
   Irritable bowel syndrome (IBS)
   Diverticulitis
   Ulcerative colitis
   Chrohn's disease
   Constipation
   Partial bowel obstruction
   Complete bowel obstruction
   Perforated duodenal ulcer
   Acute enteritis
   Colon cancer
Cardiovascular
   Leaking aortic aneurysm
   Aortic aneurysm
Other
   Pelvic adhesions
   Pelvic congestion

Chapter 2 Questions
Gynecologic and Primary Care of Women

DATA FOR ITEM 1

SB is a 22-year-old nulligravida. She comes to see you because she has not had her menstrual period in 3 months. She states that her periods are not usually very regular, but that she has never had this much time go by without a period. She also complains of fatigue and weight loss. Her physical and pelvic exams are unremarkable except for an enlarged thyroid.

1. Which of the following is the BEST first step in the management of this client?
  a. Order a thyroid panel
  b. Administer a pregnancy test
  c. Order a progesterone challenge test
  d. Refer to a gynecologist

DATA FOR ITEM 2

The following are the results of an amenorrhea workup on a 26-year-old nulligravida.

Urine hCG:	Negative
TSH:	Within normal limits
Prolactin:	Within normal limits
Progestational challenge test:	Positive withdrawal bleed following 10 days of 10 mg of Provera

2. Based on the findings above, which of the following is the MOST appropriate diagnosis for this client?
  a. Pregnancy
  b. Disorder of the hypothalamic-pituitary axis
  c. Ovarian failure
  d. Chronic anovulation

3. You would expect the levels of all of the following to be elevated during the ovulatory phase of the menstrual cycle EXCEPT:
  a. Follicle stimulation hormone (FSH)
  b. Luteinizing hormone (LH)
  c. Estrogen
  d. Progesterone

4. Which of the following is the predominant hormone of the luteal phase of the menstrual cycle?
  a. Follicle stimulation hormone (FSH)
  b. Luteinizing hormone (LH)
  c. Estrogen
  d. Progesterone

5. Which of the following statements regarding the relationship between human papillomavirus (HPV) and cervical cancer is TRUE?
  a. Approximately 40% of women with high-risk strains of HPV will develop cervical cancer.
  b. It is believed that HPV alone does not result in neoplastic changes and that co-factors to HPV infection are necessary for the development of cervical cancer.
  c. Approximately 60% to 80% of cervical cancer cases are in women with no evidence of HPV infection.
  d. Smoking doubles the risk of cervical cancer in women regardless of whether or not they are infected with HPV.

6. Which of the following classification systems for cervical cytology includes a category for benign cytology due to infections and reactive changes?
   a. The Papanicolaou System
   b. The World Health Organization System
   c. The Bethesda System (TBS)
   d. The Cervical Intraepithelial Neoplasia (CIN) System

7. How often should a 34-year-old woman who had exposure to diethylstilbestrol (DES) in utero have a Pap smear performed?
   a. Every 3 months
   b. Every 6 months
   c. Every 12 months
   d. Every 16 months

DATA FOR ITEM 8

The Pap smear results for a 34-year-old G2P1011 reveal the presence of atypical squamous cells of undetermined significance (ASCUS). Her last Pap Smear was 12 months ago and was within normal limits.

8. What is the BEST management of this client?
   a. Repeat the Pap smear in 3 to 6 months
   b. Repeat the Pap smear in 9 to 12 months
   c. Conduct or refer for colposcopy
   d. Refer to gynecologist/oncologist for biopsy and treatment

9. In which of the following regions of the cervix is cervical cancer MOST likely to begin?
   a. Cervicovaginal junction
   b. Ectocervix
   c. Endocervix
   d. Squamocolumnar junction

10. Which of the following is NOT a diagnostic criterion of premenstrual syndrome (PMS)?
   a. Symptoms that are cyclic
   b. Symptoms that last at least 3 days
   c. Symptoms that are relieved by menstruation
   d. Symptoms that interfere with activities of daily living

11. Which of the following women is MOST at risk for toxic shock syndrome (TSS)?
   a. A 34-year-old woman who uses tampons
   b. A 34-year-old woman who uses a diaphragm
   c. A 19-year-old woman who uses tampons
   d. A 19-year-old woman who uses a diaphragm

12. Unexplained recurrent or recalcitrant infections with *Candida albicans* should raise your suspicion of which of the following?
   a. HPV infection
   b. HIV infection
   c. HSV infection
   d. Bacterial vaginosis

13. Which of the following treatments for vulvovaginal candidiasis is contraindicated in pregnancy?
   a. Clotrimazole (Gyne-Lotrimin) vaginal tablet
   b. Miconazole (Monistat) vaginal suppository
   c. Fluconazole (Difulcan) oral tablet
   d. Terconazole (Terazole) vaginal cream

14. Which of the following pathogens is a causative agent of bacterial vaginosis?
    a. *Lactobacillus*
    b. *Gardneralla vaginalis*
    c. *Candida albicans*
    d. *Treponona pallidum*

15. Which of the following is the pharmacological agent of choice for treatment of bacterial vaginosis during pregnancy?
    a. Metronidazole p.o.
    b. Metronidazole vaginal gel
    c. Clindamycin p.o.
    d. Amoxicillin p.o.

16. Which of the following leads to a definitive diagnosis of trichomoniasis?
    a. Positive culture
    b. Observation of frothy, gray vaginal discharge
    c. Observation of motile trichomonads upon microscopic examination
    d. Observation of white-yellow adherent plaques on cervix and vaginal walls

17. Treatment of a woman's sexual partner(s) is indicated for all of the following infections EXCEPT:
    a. Bacterial vaginosis
    b. Trichomoniasis
    c. Gonococcal cervicitis
    d. Chlamydial infections

18. Infection with **Chlamydia trachomatis** increases your risk of all of the following EXCEPT:
    a. Premature rupture of membranes
    b. Fetal micropthalmus
    c. Infertility
    d. Ectopic pregnancy

19. Which of the following is diagnostic for infection with **Chlamydia trachomatis**?
    a. Positive cervical culture
    b. Observation of "clue cells" under microscopic examination of cervical discharge
    c. Observation of mucopurulent cervicitis
    d. Observation of increased number of white blood cells under microscopic examination of cervical discharge

20. Which of the following pharmacological agents is MOST likely to be effective in the treatment of a chlamydial infection?
    a. Benzathine penicillin IM
    b. Azithromycin p.o.
    c. Ceftriaxone IM
    d. Tetracycline p.o.

21. Which of the following pharmacological agents commonly used to treat sexually transmitted infections is NOT contraindicated for use during pregnancy?
    a. Doxycycline
    b. Tetracyline
    c. Erythromycin base
    d. Podofilox

22. Which of the following statements regarding empiric treatment of sexually transmitted infections is TRUE?

    a. Women presenting with chlamydial infection should also be treated for gonorrhea.

    b. Women presenting with chlamydial infection should also be treated for trichomoniasis.

    c. Women presenting with gonorrheal infection should also be treated for chlamydia.

    d. Women presenting with gonorrheal infection should also be treated for syphilis.

■ **DATA FOR ITEM 23**

A routine test for syphilis you ordered for a pregnant client comes back positive.

23. Which of the following management options is MOST appropriate in this situation?

    a. Watchful waiting with careful monitoring of the fetus

    b. Recommendation for a therapeutic abortion (TAB)

    c. Aggressive maternal treatment with antibiotics

    d. Aggressive neonatal treatment with antibiotics

24. Approximately what percentage of women with untreated syphilis infection experience fetal or neonatal loss?

    a. 10 %

    b. 20 %

    c. 30 %

    d. 40 %

25. Which of the following tests is diagnostic for syphilis?

    a. Positive venereal disease research laboratory (VDRL) test

    b. Positive rapid plasma reagin (RPR) test

    c. Positive darkfield microscopic examination of exudate from chancre

    d. Positive syphilis IgG antibody test

26. Which of the following criteria signals adequate treatment of syphilis?

    a. A two-fold decrease in titers

    b. A three-fold decrease in titers

    c. A four-fold decrease in titers

    d. A six-fold decrease in titers

27. What is the recommendation of the Centers for Disease Control for the treatment of a pregnant woman with syphilis who is allergic to penicillin?

    a. Wait until after pregnancy to treat

    b. Treat her with tetracycline or doxycycline

    c. Treat her with erythromycin

    d. Desensitize her to penicillin in the hospital and treat her with penicillin regimen

■ **DATA FOR ITEM 28**

As you take a medical history during an initial prenatal visit, a client reports that she suffers from occasional episodes (1 to 2 a year) of genital herpes simplex lesions. She asks you how this will affect the care you provide during pregnancy and birth.

28. Which of the following is the MOST accurate response to her question?

    a. You will treat her with Acyclovir for 7 to 10 days, which will decrease the chance of recurrent episodes of HSV lesions in pregnancy.

    b. You will start her on suppressive Acyclovir therapy at 20 weeks to decrease the frequency of recurrent episodes of HSV lesions in pregnancy.

    c. You will perform weekly cultures starting at 36 weeks of pregnancy to determine if she is having active viral shedding.

    d. You will perform a careful examination when she goes into labor or her membranes rupture, and that if she has lesions, you will recommend a cesarean section.

29. Which of the following is a clinical manifestation of infection with human papillomavirus (HPV)?
    a. Condylomata lata
    b. Condylomata acuminata
    c. Ulcerative chancre
    d. Lymphogranuloma venereum

30. Which of the following statements regarding the causative agent(s) of pelvic inflammatory disease (PID) is TRUE?
    a. Neisseria gonorrhea is the most common causative agent of PID.
    b. Chlamydia trachomatis is the most common causative agent of PID.
    c. Ascending infection due to an IUD is the most common cause of PID.
    d. Polymicrobial infection is the most common cause of PID.

31. Which of the following women can be treated on an outpatient basis for pelvic inflammatory disease (PID)?
    a. A woman who is pregnant
    b. A woman who had an IUD in place at the time of diagnosis
    c. A woman who is HIV positive
    d. A woman who you started on antibiotic treatment and has not improved in 3 days

32. Which of the following is NOT an appropriate agent in the emergency treatment of anaphylactic shock?
    a. Corticosteroids
    b. Antihistamines
    c. Epinephrine
    d. Oxygen

33. A pattern of petechiae on the cervix, a condition referred to as "strawberry cervix," is associated with which of the following infections?
    a. Candidiasis
    b. Bacterial vaginosis
    c. Trichomoniasis
    d. Gonorrheal cervicitis

34. Which of the following is the most prevalent sexually transmitted infection in the United States?
    a. Gonorrhea
    b. Chlamydia
    c. Human papillomavirus (HPV)
    d. Herpes simplex virus (HSV)

■   DATA FOR ITEM 35

A 25-year-old woman presents to your office with lower abdominal pain. The following are your findings on physical exam:

Abdominal exam:	positive abdominal guarding
Pelvic exam:	positive cervical motion tenderness, positive bilateral adenexal tenderness
Speculum exam:	positive mucopurulent discharge, increased leukocytes on wet mount

35. Based on these findings, what is the MOST likely diagnosis?
    a. Ectopic pregnancy
    b. Pelvic inflammatory disease (PID)
    c. Ruptured ovarian cyst
    d. Appendicitis

36. Which of the following is the MOST common cause of bartholinitis?
  a. Obstructed Bartholin's gland duct
  b. Physical trauma to the tissue secondary to sexual intercourse or birth
  c. Microbial infection
  d. Genetic propensity

■ **DATA FOR ITEM 37**

  On bimanual examination you note that a woman's uterus bends backwards at the isthmus.

37. How would you classify the position of this woman's uterus?
  a. Anteverted
  b. Antflexed
  c. Retroverted
  d. Retroflexed

■ **DATA FOR ITEM 38**

  FG presents to your office complaining of increased, white vaginal discharge and intense itching of her external genitalia. While performing a pelvic exam you note some white discharge with no odor and some white adherent plaques on the vaginal walls. FG's labia are excoriated as a result of scratching.

38. Which of the following is the MOST likely cause of these symptoms and of your findings?
  a. Bacterial vaginosis
  b. Candidiasis
  c. Trichomoniasis
  d. Chlamydial cervicits

■ **DATA FOR ITEM 39**

  On an annual gynecological exam you note that a client has a single, ulcerated lesion on her labia majora. She has no other symptoms or complains and states that she had not noticed or felt the lesion. The rest of her exam is unremarkable except for some inguinal lymphadenopathy.

39. Which of the following is the MOST likely cause of these findings?
  a. Primary syphilis
  b. Herpes simplex virus
  c. Chancroid
  d. Human papillomavirus

40. Which of the following is an abnormal finding on a breast examination?
  a. Clear or white discharge elicited by expression of the breast
  b. A slightly tender ridge at the caudal edge of the breast
  c. Retraction of the nipple
  d. Coarse nodularity throughout the breast

Chapter 2 Answer Key
Gynecologic and Primary Care of Women

1. *b* p. 60 PM

2. *d* p. 60 PM

3. *d* p. 5 PM

4. *d* p. 5 PM

5. *b* p. 44–45

6. *c* p. 45

7. *c* p. 46

8. *a* p. 46

9. *d* p. 781

10. *b* p. 47

11. *c* p. 48

12. *b* p. 63 PM

13. *c* p. 63 PM

14. *b* p. 50

15. *a* p. 64 PM

16. *c* p. 51

17. *a* p. 50

18. *b* p. 52

19. *a* p. 52

20. *b* p. 52

21. *c* p. 51–59

22. *c* p. 53

23. *c* p. 54–55

24. *d* p. 54

25. *c* p. 54

26. *c* p. 55

27. *d* p. 55

28. *d* p. 57

29. *b* p. 57

30. *d* p. 59

31. *b* p. 59

32. *b* p. 60

33. *c* p. 51

34. *b* p. 52

35. *b* p. 59

36. *c* p. 758, 759

37. *d* p.773–774

38. *b* p. 51

39. *a* p. 54

40. *c* p. 721–726

Chapter 3 Outline
Methods of Contraception

I.   Assisting a Client in Selecting a Method of Contraception

A. Efficacy/Effectiveness

    1. Perfect use vs. typical use failure rate

B. Safety

    1. Medical contraindications

C. Side effects

D. Cost/Convenience

E. Protection against sexually transmitted infections (STI's)/HIV

F. Permanence vs. reversibility of method/Plans for future fertility

G. Personal considerations (partner preference, frequency of intercourse, religious beliefs, etc.)

II.   Methods of Contraception

A. Abstinence

B. Natural Family Planning

    1. Ovulation method (Billings method; Creighton model)

    2. Sym–to–thermal method

    3. Calendar method

    4. Basal body temperature method

    5. Lactation amenorrhea

C. Spermicides

D. Condoms

    1. Male

    2. Female

E. Diaphragms/Cervical Caps

F. Intrauterine Contraceptive Devices

    1. Copper T 380A (ParaGard)

    2. Progesterone T (Progestasert)

G. Oral Hormonal Contraception

    1. Combination oral contraceptives

    2. Progestin-only pill/Minipill

        i. Monthly Combination Contraceptive Injection (Lunelle)

H. Depot-medroxyprogesterone acetate (DMPA)/(Depo-Provera)

I. Subdermal Levonorgestrel Implants (Norplant)

J. Sterilization

K. Emergency Contraception
  1. Mifepristone (RU–486)

Know the following for each of the above methods of contraception:

A. Mechanism(s) of Action

B. Efficacy/Effectiveness

C. Indications/Advantages

D. Disadvantages/Cautions

E. Contraindications

F. Side effects
  1. Positive
  2. Negative

G. Warning signs

H. Instructions for starting and using method (if applicable)

I. Technique for inserting/administering method (if applicable)

J. Managing side effects/complications

III. Management of Special Circumstances

A. Unintended pregnancy while using a method of contraception

B. Use of contraceptives while breastfeeding

C. Latex allergies/allergies to spermicides

D. Missed oral contraceptive pills

E. Missed DMPA shots

F. Missing IUD strings

G. Drug interactions

H. Desired pregnancy/Return to fertility

I. Back-up methods of contraception

Chapter 3 Questions
Methods of Contraception

1. Of the following natural family planning (NFP) methods, which is the MOST effective?
   a. The sympto-thermal method
   b. The calendar/rhythm method
   c. The basal body temperature method
   d. The cervical mucus method

▪ **DATA FOR ITEM 2**

   KH has been keeping a record of her menstrual cycles for the last 12 months because she wants to use the calendar method as her method of family planning. You have explained, and she understands, the limits of this method. Her cycle lengths have been as follows: 27 days, 27 days, 30 days, 26 days, 30 days, 28 days, 27 days, 27 days, 30 days, 28 days, 26 days, 27 days.

2. According to the guidelines for the calendar method, what is KH's period of fertility?
   a. Day 10 to day 16 of her menstrual cycle
   b. Day 6 to day 20 of her menstrual cycle
   c. Day 12 to day 22 of her menstrual cycle
   d. Day 16 to day 20 of her menstrual cycle

3. The changes in cervical mucus that make the ovulation/cervical mucus/Billing's method of family planning possible are MOSTLY due to which of the following?
   a. Estrogen
   b. Progesterone
   c. Gonadotropin releasing hormone (GnRH)
   d. Prostaglandins

4. In order to avoid pregnancy, the woman using the cervical mucus method of family planning should avoid intercourse for a minimum of how many days following the "peak day" of her cycle?
   a. 2 days
   b. 3 days
   c. 4 days
   d. 5 days

5. The basal body temperature method by itself can only determine which of the following?
   a. When ovulation has occurred
   b. When ovulation will occur
   c. Pre-ovulatory fertile and infertile days
   d. When the next menstrual period will occur

6. Which of the following statements about the lactation amenorrhea method (LAM) is TRUE?
   a. When the guidelines for its use are followed, it is 98% effective in preventing pregnancy.
   b. Even when the guidelines for its use are followed, it is only 30% to 40% effective in preventing pregnancy.
   c. It is effective for up to 9–12 months following birth as long as the infant is exclusively breast-feeding.
   d. It is based on the inhibition of ovulation caused by progesterone.

7. Which of the following statements about nonoxynol–9 is FALSE?

    a. It is the active ingredient in most spermicidal preparations and is available without a prescription.

    b. In the laboratory, nonoxynol–9 is lethal to the agents that cause gonorrhea, trichomoniasis, syphilis, chlamydia, and AIDS.

    c. It lowers the chance of becoming infected with a bacterial sexually transmitted disease.

    d. It lowers the chance of becoming infected with the human immunodeficiency virus (HIV).

8. Which of the following statements would indicate that a woman has understood how to properly use a spermicidal agent?

    a. "I need to wait 4 hours after the last time I have sex before I can use a douche."

    b. "I need to wait 30 minutes after I insert the spermicide for it to become effective."

    c. "If I do not have sex within 1 hour of inserting the spermicide, I need to reapply the spermicide."

    d. "I am protected for 1 hour after insertion of the spermicide even if I have sex more than once in that hour."

9. Which of the following statements regarding condoms is TRUE?

    a. Only latex, not lambskin or polyurethane, condoms protect both against sexually transmitted diseases and pregnancy.

    b. Latex condoms are only effective at preventing transmission of sexually transmitted diseases if they have a spermicidal lubricant.

    c. Unlike latex condoms, polyurethane condoms are safe to use with any type of lubricant including oil-based lubricants.

    d. Lambskin condoms protect against pregnancy and bacterial sexually transmitted diseases but not against viral sexually transmitted diseases.

10. Which of the following should NOT be included in your instructions regarding the proper use of condoms?

    a. Leave a $\frac{1}{2}$ inch space at the end of a plain-tipped condom

    b. Check for holes/leakage by filling the condom with water or air

    c. Ensure that there is adequate lubrication on the exterior of the condom

    d. Following ejaculation, the male must withdraw while still erect and while holding the rim of the condom

11. The female condom is made of which of the following materials?

    a. Rubber

    b. Polyurethane

    c. Latex

    d. Lambskin

12. Which of the following statements about the female condom is TRUE?

    a. It comes in different sizes and has to be fitted by a health care professional.

    b. It should be used without any lubrication to ensure that it remains in place.

    c. It is more expensive than the male condom, but it can be reused.

    d. It offers a high rate of protection against HIV, herpes simplex, gonorrhea, and chlamydia.

13. What is the minimum amount of time after the last act of intercourse that a woman must leave a diaphragm in position in order to maximize contraceptive effectiveness?

    a. 2 hours

    b. 4 hours

    c. 6 hours

    d. 8 hours

14. If a diaphragm is properly cared for and remains a proper fit, for how long is it usable?
    a. 1 year
    b. 2 years
    c. 3 years
    d. 4 years

15. Which of the following statements indicates that a woman has understood how to properly care for and store her diaphragm?
    a. "I should soak my diaphragm in a 10% bleach solution and then rinse it and dry it thoroughly before storing it in a dry container."
    b. "I should wash my diaphragm with an antibacterial soap, rinse thoroughly, apply some talcum powder or cornstarch to keep it dry, and store in a dry container."
    c. "I should wash my diaphragm with a mild soap, rinse and dry thoroughly, and then store in a dry container."
    d. "I should wash my diaphragm with a mild soap, rinse and dry thoroughly, apply some petroleum jelly to avoid cracking, and store in a dry place."

16. Which of the following statements regarding the effectiveness of diaphragms is FALSE?
    a. With typical use, the diaphragm has a failure rate of approximately 18%.
    b. The frequency of intercourse significantly affects the effectiveness of the diaphragm among women who are consistent diaphragm users.
    c. The use of a spermicide significantly increases the effectiveness of the diaphragm.
    d. The majority of cases of diaphragm failure are due to lack of patient diligence or lack of ability by women to understand the proper technique to use the diaphragm.

▮ DATA FOR ITEM 17

A 32-year-old G2P1011 desires to use a diaphragm as her method of contraception. She has successfully used a coil spring diaphragm prior to the birth of her child. During her pelvic exam you determine that her uterus is retroverted, that the arch behind her symphysis pubis is average, and that she has a first-degree cystocele.

17. Which of the following is the MOST appropriate choice for this woman?
    a. A coil spring diaphragm
    b. An arcing spring diaphragm
    c. A method other than a diaphragm

18. Which of the following is the correct set of instructions regarding the proper use of a spermicide with a diaphragm?
    a. Before inserting the diaphragm, evenly spread approximately one teaspoon of spermicide around the inside of the cup and the rim of the diaphragm. For a repeat act of intercourse, remove the diaphragm and repeat the steps above.
    b. Before inserting the diaphragm, evenly spread approximately one teaspoon of spermicide around the rim and inside of the cup. For a repeat act of intercourse, insert an applicator-full of spermicide without removing the diaphragm.
    c. After inserting the diaphragm, insert one applicator-full of spermicide before intercourse begins. For a repeat act of intercourse, insert another applicator-full of spermicide without removing the diaphragm.

19. Which of the following statements about the cervical cap is TRUE?
    a. The cervical cap is as effective for parous as it is for nulliparous women.
    b. The cervical cap, like the diaphragm, can be used during menstruation.
    c. With the cervical cap, additional spermicide is not needed for repeated acts of intercourse.
    d. The cervical cap should be removed 24 hours after insertion.

20. Research has indicated that which of the following statements most accurately describes the MOST likely mechanism of action for the Copper T 30A (ParaGard) intrauterine contraceptive device (IUD)?

    a. It prevents implantation of a fertilized ovum by creating a hostile uterine environment.

    b. It releases progesterone, which affects fallopian tube motility and alters the uterine lining.

    c. It prevents fertilization from occurring by altering fallopian tube motility and incapacitating the sperm.

    d. It acts as a physical and mechanical barrier to the fallopian tubes, thus blocking the sperm from reaching the ovum.

21. Which of the following is NOT an absolute contraindication for the insertion of an IUD?

    a. Recurrent pelvic inflammatory disease (PID)

    b. Nulliparity

    c. Genital actinomycosis

    d. Cervical stenosis

22. How long after insertion must the Progesterone T (Progestasert) intrauterine device (IUD) be replaced in order to remain effective?

    a. 1 year

    b. 2 years

    c. 5 to 7 years

    d. 10 years

23. At what point during the menstrual cycle should an intrauterine device be inserted?

    a. During menstruation when the cervical os is slightly dilated and the risk of inserting the IUD into a pregnant uterus is eliminated

    b. Mid-cycle so that the risk of infection is reduced as long as pregnancy can be precluded

    c. During the first seven days of the cycle to reduce the risk of inserting the IUD into a pregnant uterus

    d. Anytime of the cycle as long as pregnancy and vaginitis/cervicitis can be precluded

24. Which of the following is NOT a prerequisite to the insertion of an intrauterine device (IUD)?

    a. Informed consent form signed by the woman

    b. Pregnancy test

    c. Chlamydia and gonorrhea cultures

    d. Pap smear

■ DATA FOR ITEMS 25–26

TR, a 33-year-old G3P2012 comes to see you because she has missed her period and she thinks she may be pregnant. She had an IUD inserted 2 years ago and has never had any problems with it. TR states that if she is pregnant, she and her husband desire to continue with the pregnancy. You perform a pregnancy test that comes back positive. Upon speculum examination, you can visualize the IUD strings protruding from the cervical os.

25. Which of the following is the MOST appropriate management of this situation?

    a. Leave the IUD in place because there is a high chance of inducing an abortion during a removal of the IUD

    b. Remove the IUD immediately in order to reduce the risk of infection and abortion

    c. Obtain an ultrasound to determine the position of the IUD before deciding whether to leave the IUD in or to remove it

    d. Refer the woman for medical management

26. You know that TR is at increased risk for all of the following EXCEPT:
    a. Sepsis
    b. Placenta previa
    c. Placenta accreta
    d. Ectopic pregnancy

27. Which of the following is the most appropriate first management step of a client with missing IUD strings whom you have determined is not pregnant?
    a. Using sterile instruments and technique, search the cervical canal for the IUD or the IUD strings
    b. Obtain an ultrasound to determine if the IUD is in the uterus or whether is has been expelled
    c. Recommend that the woman obtain an x-ray to rule-out uterine perforation/migration of the IUD into the abdominal cavity
    d. Insert another IUD if the woman desires to continue with the same method

■   **DATA FOR ITEM 28**

    A client who has an IUD in place has determined that she desires another pregnancy.

28. Which of the following MOST appropriately describes the proper procedure for removal of the IUD in a woman with visible/palpable IUD strings?
    a. Instruct the woman to wait for her next menses and to follow the same procedure she does to check for her IUD strings, but that this time she should grasp and gently pull on the strings to remove the IUD. Tell her that if the IUD does not come out easily, she should come in to have you remove it.
    b. Have the woman come in to see you and, using a long-handled forceps or a needle-holder, exert steady but gentle traction to remove the IUD
    c. Have the woman come in to see you and, using alligator forceps, find the IUD within the uterine cavity and grasp it with the forceps. Pull evenly and steadily with the forceps to remove it.
    d. Refer the woman for IUD removal under ultrasound guidance

29. Following the initial visit at 3 to 6 weeks following the IUD insertion, how often should a woman with no problems be seen by a health care provider for a physical, pelvic exam, and pap smear?
    a. Every 2 to 3 months
    b. Every 6 months
    c. Every 8 months
    d. Every 12 months

30. Which of the following terms is used to describe the type of oral hormonal contraception in which the same amount of estrogen and progestin are taken each day for 20 to 21 days followed by 7 days of no hormonal intake?
    a. Monophasic
    b. Biphasic
    c. Triphasic
    d. Minipill

31. Which of the following BEST describes the main mechanism of action of the combination oral contraceptive pill to prevent pregnancy?
    a. Modification of fallopian tube motility, which affects speed of ovum transport
    b. Supression of ovulation by suppression of follicle-stimulating hormone (FSH) and luteinizing hormone (LH)
    c. Creation of an atrophic endometrium that is hostile to implantation by a fertilized ovum
    d. Inhibition of sperm capacitation

32. Which of the following is the synthetic estrogen that is used in combination oral contraceptives with less than 50 mcg of estrogen?

    a. Mestranol
    b. Ethinyl estradiol
    c. Levonogesterel
    d. Norethindrone

33. Which of the following is the progestin that is used as the index progestin in order to compare the biological potency of the various progestins used in oral contraceptives?

    a. Mestranol
    b. Ethinyl estradiol
    c. Levonogesterel
    d. Norethindrone

34. Which of the following is NOT an absolute contraindication to the use of oral hormonal contraception?

    a. Presence or history of thrombophlebitis
    b. Smoking by women over the age of 35
    c. Classic migraine headaches with aura
    d. Undiagnosed abnormal genital bleeding

35. Which of the following statements regarding the link of oral contraceptives and reproductive cancers is TRUE?

    a. Oral contraceptives significantly increase a woman's overall lifetime risk of developing breast cancer.
    b. Oral contraceptives significantly increase the risk of endometrial cancer.
    c. Oral contraceptives significantly decreases the risk of ovarian cancer.
    d. Oral contraceptives significantly decrease the risk of cervical cancer.

36. Which of the following is NOT a prerequisite to prescribing an oral contraceptive for a client?

    a. Obtaining informed consent
    b. Conducting a pelvic examination that includes a pap
    c. Screening for any deviations from normal or contraindications for the use of oral contraceptive pills
    d. Providing instructions on taking oral contraceptive pills

37. Which of the following BEST describes the reasoning for delaying the initiation of combination oral contraceptives in a postpartum woman who is not breastfeeding?

    a. Because earlier initiation of combination oral contraceptives can interfere with adequate involution of the uterus
    b. Because earlier initiation of combination oral contraceptives can interfere with adequate initiation of breastfeeding
    c. Because earlier initiation of combination oral contraceptives can increase the risk of thromboembolism
    d. Because earlier initiation of combination oral contraceptives can increase the risk of delayed postpartum hemorrhage

38. How soon after a first-term abortion can a woman safely start taking combination oral contraceptives?

    a. Immediately
    b. 1 week
    c. 3 weeks
    d. 6 weeks

39. Which of the following advice is MOST appropriate to give a postpartum woman who is exclusively breastfeeding and who desires oral contraception?
   a. Combination oral contraceptives are most effective, so she should wait for 6 weeks and then initiate combination oral contraceptives
   b. Combination oral contraceptives are most effective, but that she should start with the mini-pill in the immediate postpartum period, and then switch to combination oral contraceptives at 6 weeks postpartum
   c. That the mini-pill is the oral contraceptive of choice for breastfeeding women, and that she should start with the mini-pill in the immediate postpartum period
   d. That the mini-pill is the oral contraceptive of choice for breastfeeding women, and that she can start safely taking the mini-pill at approximately 4–6 weeks postpartum

40. Which of the following symptoms should be reported immediately by a woman who is taking oral contraceptives?
   a. Nausea and vomiting
   b. Hemopytsis
   c. Mood changes
   d. Breakthrough bleeding/spotting

41. To ensure maximal contraceptive effectiveness and minimize the chances of breakthrough bleeding, when in a woman's cycle should oral contraception be started?
   a. Within the first five days of the cycle
   b. Within the first ten days of the cycle
   c. Mid-cycle
   d. Within the last ten days of the cycle

42. For at least how long should a woman use back-up contraception if she has missed two of her combination oral contraceptive pills?
   a. 7 days
   b. 14 days
   c. For the rest of the current pill packet
   d. For a full cycle (28 days)

DATA FOR ITEM 43

LG is a client whom you started on a combination oral contraceptive 2 months ago. Today she calls to tell you that she is having some breakthrough bleeding. She has taken her pills everyday as instructed. She states she has to use a sanitary napkin, but that the bleeding is less than she has during her menstrual periods. She has no pain or cramping and her last menstrual period was normal. She had breakthrough bleeding with her first pill cycle as well.

43. What is the MOST appropriate action to take at this time?
   a. Recommend that she use a back-up method until the bleeding has stopped, and reassure her that in most cases breakthrough bleeding will remit by her fourth pill-cycle
   b. Have her come in to your office so that you can perform an exam and rule out pregnancy
   c. Have her come in to your office so that you can switch her to another pill or start her on a new contraceptive method
   d. Have her come in to your office so that you can switch her to a non-hormonal method of contraception

44. If a woman using the combination oral contraceptive pill is having breakthrough bleeding and spotting in the early half of the cycle (pill days 1 to 9), the bleeding is MOST likely due to which of the following?

a. Estrogen excess

b. Estrogen deficiency

c. Progestin excess

d. Progestin deficiency

45. Which of the following CANNOT be used as a method of emergency contraception?

a. Combination oral contraceptives

b. Progestin-only oral contraceptives

c. Depo-provera

d. IUD's

46. What is the maximum amount of time after an unprotected act of intercourse that the Yupze regimen of oral contraceptive pills is considered to be effective as a method of emergency contraception?

a. 24 hours

b. 48 hours

c. 72 hours

d. 96 hours

47. What is the maximum amount of time after an act of unprotected of intercourse that a copper-releasing IUD is considered to be effective as a method of emergency contraception?

a. 72 hours

b. 96 hours

c. 5 to 7 days

d. 7 to 14 days

48. What is the MOST common side effect of the Yupze regimen of combination oral contraceptives used as emergency contraception?

a. Headache

b. Bleeding

c. Nausea/vomiting

d. Menstrual irregularities

DATA FOR ITEM 49

MN is a 30-year-old who has just started taking combination oral contraceptive pills. She is in to see you for her 3-month pill check. She states that she has been having migraine headaches with vision changes. She did not suffer from migraine headaches previous to initiating the pill.

49. Which of the following is the MOST appropriate management of this client?

a. Send her for a consult with a neurologist since the migraine headaches are unlikely to be related to the oral contraceptive pill

b. Reassure her that most side effects remit on their own by the fourth pill cycle. Have her continue taking the pill and have her come in for a follow-up visit in one month

c. Switch her to another combination oral contraceptive pill that is less likely to cause this side effect. Schedule her for a follow-up visit in 3 months

d. Switch her to a method of contraception that does not contain estrogen or to a non-hormonal method of contraception

50. Which of the following BEST describes Depo-Provera's main mechanism of action?
   a. Modification of fallopian tube motility, which affects speed of ovum transport
   b. Suppression of ovulation by suppression of follicle-stimulating hormone (FSH) and luteinizing hormone (LH)
   c. Creation of an atrophic endometrium that is hostile to implantation by a fertilized ovum
   d. Thickening of the cervical mucus, which prevents passage of sperm

51. Which of the following is the MOST common side effect of Depo-Provera?
   a. Headaches
   b. Menstrual changes
   c. Weight gain
   d. Mood changes

52. Which of the following statements about Depo-Provera is TRUE?
   a. It has a quick return of fertility post discontinuation.
   b. It is protective against pelvic inflammatory disease.
   c. It increased the frequency of seizures in women with seizure disorders.
   d. It increases the risk of endometrial cancer.

53. How soon after birth can a woman who is breastfeeding initiate Depo-Provera?
   a. Within 5 days of delivery
   b. 2 weeks postpartum
   c. 4 weeks postpartum
   d. 6 weeks postpartum

54. How often should a woman be scheduled to receive her injection of Depo-Provera?
   a. Every 10 weeks
   b. Every 12 weeks
   c. Every 14 weeks
   d. Every 16 weeks

55. When does Depo-Provera become effective if a woman receives her first injection within 5 days of the beginning of her menstruation?
   a. Immediately
   b. 48 hours
   c. 5 days
   d. 7 days

56. Which of the following is the MOST effective contraceptive method?
   a. Depo-Provera
   b. Norplant
   c. Female sterilization
   d. Male sterilization

57. How soon after insertion does Norplant become effective in preventing pregnancy?
   a. 12 hours
   b. 24 to 48 hours
   c. 72 to 96 hours
   d. 7 days

58. Which of the following side effects is MOST commonly cited as a reason for the discontinuation of Norplant?
   a. Weight gain
   b. Headaches
   c. Menstrual changes
   d. Breast tenderness

59. Which of the following is the MOST popular method of birth control in the United States?

    a. The combination oral contraceptive pill

    b. The condom

    c. Depo-Provera

    d. Sterilization

DATA FOR ITEM 60

FB is a 35-year-old G4P3013 who smokes ½ pack of cigarettes a day and desires a highly effective method of contraception to use until her husband gets a vasectomy in approximately 3 months. She does not desire any more children. She has no allergies to latex and has no contraindication to the use of hormonal contraceptive methods.

60. Which of the following methods of contraception is MOST appropriate for FB?

    a. Combination oral contraceptives

    b. Diaphragm

    c. Depo-provera

    d. Condoms

DATA FOR ITEM 61

HJ is a 25-year-old G2P2002 who is in to see you for her 6 week postpartum visit. She is breastfeeding and plans to continue to do so for at least 6 months, but possibly for longer. She and her husband desire an effective method of birth control that HJ can use long-term, but that is reversible because they are unsure about whether or not they will want to have another baby in the future. In the past LH has used combination oral contraceptives and condoms with spermicide, but she states that the spermicide irritated her and caused her to have yeast infections so she stopped using it. Her medical and family history is unremarkable.

61. Which of the following methods of contraception is MOST appropriate for HJ?

    a. Diaphragm

    b. Intrauterine device

    c. Combination oral contraceptives

    d. Cervical cap

DATA FOR ITEM 62

SD is a 27-year-old G3P1111 who comes to see you to initiate a method of contraception. She has an infant that is 11 months old and she hopes to have another child in 1–2 years. Her history is remarkable for a deep venous thrombosis (DVT) that developed during her first pregnancy. Her physical and pelvic exams today are within normal limits.

62. Which of the following methods of contraception is MOST appropriate for SD?

    a. Diaphragm

    b. Cervical cap

    c. Combination oral contraceptive

    d. Norplant

Chapter 3 Answer Key
Methods of Contraception

1. *a* p. 73	**22.** *a* p. 103	**43.** *a* p. 121
2. *b* p. 74	**23.** *d* p. 104	**44.** *b* p. 118, 121
3. *a* p. 74	**24.** *b* p. 104	**45.** *c* p. 124 –125
4. *b* p. 75	**25.** *b* p. 109	**46.** *c* p. 125
5. *a* p. 76	**26.** *c* p. 109	**47.** *c* p. 125
6. *a* p. 78	**27.** *a* p. 109–110	**48.** *c* p. 125
7. *d* p. 83	**28.** *b* p. 110	**49.** *d* p. 116–121
8. *c* p. 85	**29.** *d* p. 111	**50.** *b* p. 127
9. *c* p. 87	**30.** *a* p. 113	**51.** *b* p. 128
10. *b* p. 86–87	**31.** *b* p. 113	**52.** *b* p. 128
11. *b* p. 87	**32.** *b* p. 114	**53.** *d* p. 129
12. *d* p. 88	**33.** *d* p. 114	**54.** *b* p. 129
13. *c* p. 91	**34.** *b* p. 116	**55.** *a* p. 127
14. *b* p. 91	**35.** *c* p. 117, 119	**56.** *b* p. 68, 129
15. *c* p. 96	**36.** *b* p. 119	**57.** *b* p. 129
16. *d* p. 92	**37.** *c* p. 120	**58.** *c* p. 130
17. *c* p. 93	**38.** *a* p. 120	**59.** *d* p. 69
18. *b* p. 96	**39.** *d* p. 120	**60.** *c*
19. *c* p. 97–99	**40.** *b* p. 122	**61.** *b*
20. *c* p. 101	**41.** *a* p. 120	**62.** *a*
21. *b* p. 102	**42.** *a* p. 122	

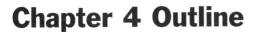

Chapter 4 Outline

Care of the Perimenopausal/Postmenopausal Woman

I.   Definition of Menopause

II. Physiology of Menopause

Changes in hormonal levels (FSH/LH assessments)

III. Diagnosing Menopause

IV. Discomforts/Sequelae of Menopause

- Menstrual irregularities
- Sleep disturbances
- Hot flashes
- Vaginal atrophy
- Dyspareunia
- Urinary incontinence
- Cardiovascular disease
- Osteoporosis
- Changes in cognitive function
- Skin changes

Know the following for each of the above discomforts:

A. Etiology

B. Signs/Symptoms

C. Management/Treatment

V.   Hormone Replacement Therapy

A. Regimens

B. Indications/Contraindications

C. Side effects

VI. Preventive Health Screening

A. Urinalysis/Urine dipstick

B. Pap smear (with optional maturation index or cornification count)

C. Mammography

D. Occult stool test

E. Fasting plasma cholesterol and triglycerides/lipid profile

F. Colonoscopy

VII.   Pelvic and Breast Masses in the Postmenopausal Woman

VIII.   Management of Uterine Bleeding in the Postmenopausal Woman

IX.   Contraceptive Needs of the Perimenopausal Woman

Chapter 4 Questions

Care of the Perimenopausal and Postmenopausal Woman

1. What is the average age of menopause among women in the United States?
   a. 49
   b. 50
   c. 51
   d. 52

2. Which of the following BEST describes the reason for the increased risk of endometrial cancer seen with estrogen replacement therapy (ERT)?
   a. Excessive estrogen doses
   b. Unopposed estrogen
   c. Unopposed progesterone
   d. Use of the wrong synthetic estrogen

3. Which of the following is the characteristic hormonal change of perimenopause (6 to 7 years before menopause)?
   a. Increased level of follicle stimulating hormone (FSH)
   b. Increased level of luteinizing hormone (LH)
   c. Decreased level of estradiol
   d. Increased level of inhibin

4. Which of the following estrogens is predominant in the postmenopausal period?
   a. Ethinyl estradiol
   b. Estriol
   c. Estrone
   d. Estradiol

5. MOST women entering menopause will experience which of the following menstrual cycle changes?
   a. Sudden amenorrhea
   b. Oligomenorrhea or hypomenorrhea
   c. Menorrhagia
   d. Hypermenorrhea

■ DATA FOR ITEM 6

   A 54-year-old woman has come to see you because after 20 months of amenorrhea she is now experiencing some bleeding. On pelvic exam you note that there is no apparent vaginal or cervical source for the bleeding.

6. What is the MOST appropriate assessment and management of this situation?
   a. This type of sporadic bleeding is a normal occurrence up to 24 months following the cessation of menses that is associated with menopause. Follow-up with the woman in 4 to 6 months.
   b. This type of sporadic bleeding is a normal occurrence up to 24 months following the cessation of menses that is associated with menopause. Order cervical cultures and a pap smear to rule out infection/pre-cancerous cervical changes.
   c. It is rare for vaginal bleeding to recur after 12 months of amenorrhea. Order a work-up for organic disease that includes an endometrial biopsy.
   d. It is rare for vaginal bleeding to recur after 12 months of amenorrhea. Order an ultrasound to assess endometrial thickness.

7. Which of the following physiological changes seen in menopausal women is NOT related to decreased estrogen?
   a. Thinning of the vaginal epithelium
   b. Atrophic endometrium
   c. Loss of elasticity of the skin
   d. Loss of bone density

8. Menopause is NOT statistically associated with an increase in which of the following?
   a. Hot flashes
   b. Clinical depression
   c. Sleep disturbances
   d. Atrophic changes of the reproductive tract

9. Which of the following is NOT a benign skin change?
   a. Seborrheic keratosis
   b. Cherry angioma
   c. Melanoma
   d. Fibroepithelioma

10. Which of the following is the MOST common symptom associated with menopause?
    a. Irritability
    b. Hot flashes
    c. Fatigue
    d. Urinary frequency

11. How often should a woman over the age of 50 have a routine screening mammogram?
    a. Every 3 years
    b. Every 2 years
    c. Every year
    d. Every 6 months

◼ DATA FOR ITEM 12

A 59-year-old woman who is considering hormone replacement therapy (HRT) asks you about the connection between HRT and breast cancer.

12. Which of the following answers to this question would be MOST accurate?
    a. There is no conclusive evidence that a woman's overall risk of breast cancer is increased by hormone replacement therapy (HRT).
    b. HRT has been demonstrated to significantly increase a woman's lifetime risk of developing breast cancer.
    c. The addition of progestin to hormone replacement therapy has been shown to decrease the risk of breast cancer for women on HRT.
    d. The risk of developing breast cancer due to HRT is related both to the duration and the dose of estrogen.

13. What is the leading cause of death for postmenopausal women in the United States?
    a. Lung cancer
    b. Breast cancer
    c. Cardiovascular disease
    d. Respiratory diseases and infection

14. Which of the following is NOT a risk factor for osteoporosis?
    a. Thin or small body frame
    b. Sedentary lifestyle
    c. Family history
    d. African-American descent

15. Estrogen therapy reduces the risk of fractures by approximately what percent?
    a. 20%
    b. 30%
    c. 40%
    d. 50%

16. Which of the following therapeutic measures has NOT been demonstrated to decrease the risk of bone fracture in postmenopausal women?
    a. Addition of vitamin D to the diet
    b. Addition of calcium to the diet
    c. Weight-bearing exercise
    d. Estrogen replacement therapy

17. What is the minimum daily dose of conjugated estrogen that is effective in maintaining bone mass?
    a. 0.05 mg
    b. 0.3 mg
    c. 0.625 mg
    d. 1.0 mg

18. For which of the following women would an endometrial biopsy be MOST indicated?
    a. A 65-year-old woman who has been on hormone replacement therapy for 10 years
    b. A 58-year-old woman who is on sequential/cyclical hormone therapy who has uterine bleeding on day 21 of each month
    c. A 60-year-old woman who has been on the continuous hormone replacement therapy (HRT), Prempro, for 2 years and is experiencing uterine bleeding
    d. A 52-year-old woman who has been on continuous hormone replacement therapy (HRT), Prempro, for 2 months and is experiencing uterine bleeding

19. Which of the following is the hormone used to confirm the onset of menopause?
    a. Serum FSH level
    b. Serum LH level
    c. Serum estradiol level
    d. Serum estrone level

20. Which of the following is the correct standard dose for continuous hormone replacement therapy (HRT)?
    a. 0.625 mg conjugated estrogens (Premarin) daily; 2.5 mg medroxyprogesterone (Provera) daily
    b. 0.625 mg conjugated estrogens (Premarin) daily; 5–10 mg medroxyprogesterone (Provera) daily
    c. 0.625 mg estrogen (Premarin) daily; 5–10 mg medroxyprogesterone (Provera) in the first 2 weeks of the month
    d. 0.625 mg estrogen (Premarin) on days 1–25; 2.5 mg medroxyprogesterone (Provera) on days 12 through 25

Chapter 4 Answer Key
Care of the Perimenopausal and Postmenopausal Woman

1. *c* p. 202

2. *b* p. 203

3. *a* p. 204

4. *c* p. 205

5. *b* p. 205

6. *c* p. 205

7. *c* p. 208

8. *b* p. 206

9. *c* p. 210

10. *b* p. 206

11. *c* p. 211

12. *a* p. 211

13. *c* p. 211–212

14. *d* p. 212–213

15. *d* p. 214

16. *a* p. 213

17. *c* p. 218

18. *c* p. 219–220

19. *a* p. 201, 215

20. *a* p. 219

Chapter 5 Outline

Care of the HIV-Infected Woman and Other Special Primary Care Situations

I.   Care of the HIV-Infected Woman

A. Pathophysiology of HIV infection

B. Transmission and Epidemiology

C. Diagnosis/Laboratory Testing

    1. HIV antibody tests

        a. Enzyme immunoassay (EIA) or Enzyme-linked immunosorbent assay (ELISA)

        b. Western blot

        c. Viral Culture

        d. Polymerase chain reaction (PCR)

        e. P24 antigen assays

    2. HIV Counseling and Education

        a. Preventive counseling and education

        b. Pre- and post-test counseling

        c. HIV counseling and testing of pregnant women

        d. Partner notification

        e. Confidentiality/Informed consent issues

    3. Clinical Manifestations of HIV infection/AIDS

        a. Eye/visual abnormalities

        b. Candidiasis (oral and vaginal)

        c. Low grade/Persistent fever

        d. Lymph node enlargement

        e. Rashes/Skin lesions

        f. HPV infection/Genital warts/Invasive cervical cancer

        g. Weight loss/Intractable diarrhea

        h. Pneumonia

    4. Assessment of Immune Status

        a. Viral load

        b. CD4 cell counts

    5. Special Screening/Immunization Needs

        a. CBC

        b. Tuberculosis

        c. Anergy panel

        d. STI screening (including syphilis)

        e. Hepatitis panel

        f. Liver enzyme tests

        g. Toxoplasmosis titer

        h. Tetanus, Hepatitis B, Pneumovax, and Influenza immunizations

6. Contraceptive/Safer Sex Needs

7. Management and Treatment of HIV Disease

    a. Antiretroviral therapy

        i. Drug regimens/Combination therapies

        ii. Management of drug side effects/complications

        iii. Monitoring of therapy effectiveness

8. Treatment of opportunistic infections

9. HIV Infection in Pregnancy

    a. HIV counseling and testing of pregnant women

    b. Care of the HIV-infected pregnant woman

        i. Case management/coordination of social services

        ii. Co-management with primary care provider

        iii. Treatment/management of substance abuse

        iv. Labs

        v. Assessment of immune status

        vi. Monitoring of drug therapy effectiveness

        vii. Management of drug therapy side effects

        viii. Screening and treatment of STI's/opportunistic infections

    c. Reducing perinatal/vertical transmission and management of the HIV-infected woman in labor and birth

        i. The AIDS Clinical Trial Group Protocol 076

        ii. Pregnancy and intrapartum zidovudine treatment protocols

        iii. Other pregnancy and intrapartum treatment protocols

        iv. Obstetric interventions (internal fetal monitoring, fetal scalp blood sampling, AROM) and vertical transmission

        v. Vaginal vs. Cesarean Section birth

        vi. Management of premature rupture of membranes (PROM) in the HIV-infected woman

    d. Management and treatment of infants born to HIV-infected women

        i. HIV testing of the neonate

        ii. Antiretroviral treatment of the neonate

10. Universal Precautions

II. Care of the Lesbian/Bisexual Client

A. Effects of homophobia on the health status and health-seeking behaviors of lesbian/bisexual clients.

B. Cervical Cancer Screening for the Lesbian/Bisexual Client

C. Contraceptive Needs of the Lesbian/Bisexual Client

D. Safer Sex Needs of the Lesbian/Bisexual Client

E. The Lesbian/Bisexual Client and HIV/AIDS

F. The Lesbian/Bisexual Client or Couple and Childbearing

G. The Lesbian/Bisexual Client and Domestic Violence and/or Rape

III. Care of the Substance Abusing Woman

A. Definitions
  1. Abuse
  2. Dependence
  3. Addiction
  4. Tolerance

• Caffeine

• Tobacco

• Alcohol

• Marijuana

• Cocaine/Crack

• Amphetamines

• Opiates (morphine, codeine, meperidine, fentanyl, heroin, methadone, oxymorphone, and hydromorphone)

Know the following for each of the above substances:

B. Signs/Symptoms of Abuse

C. Side Effects/Complications

D. Fetal Effects/Impact on Pregnancy of Maternal Substance Abuse
  1. Signs of drug exposure in the newborn

E. Management of Abuse/Treatment of Addiction

F. Management of Abuse in Pregnancy and/or Lactation

G. Dual-Diagnosis Disorders

IV. Care of the Adolescent Client

A. Definition and Physiology of Puberty
  1. Thelarche (Breast development)
  2. Genital Development
  3. Menarche
  4. Tanner Staging System

B. Examination of the Adolescent Client

C. Abnormalities of Pubescence
  1. Amenorrhea (Primary vs. Secondary)
  2. Precocious Puberty
  3. Delayed Puberty

V Domestic Violence

A. Definition

B. Signs/Symptoms

C. Screening/Safety Assessment

D. Intervention, Management, and Referral
1. Documentation of findings
2. Reporting responsibilities of the clinician
3. Crisis counseling

E. Violence During Pregnancy

VI   Rape/Sexual Assault

A. Definition

B. Signs/Symptoms

C. Screening/Safety Assessment

D. Intervention, Management, and Referral
1. The post-rape/sexual assault examination
   a. Use of evidence collection protocol
2. Emergency contraception
3. STI screening/Use of antibiotic or antiretroviral prophylaxis
4. Crisis counseling
5. Reporting responsibilities of the clinician/Collaboration with police

VII   Sexual Counseling/Sexual Dysfunction

A. Taking a Sexual History

B. Sexual Dysfunctions
1. Dyspareunia
2. Inhibited sexual desire
3. Vaginismus
4. Anorgasmia
5. Vulvodynia
   a. Definition
   b. Etiology
   c. Signs/Symptoms
   d. Management/Treatment

VIII   Out-of-Hospital Birth

A. Definitions and Models
1. Birth Centers
2. Home Births

B. Characteristics and Principles of Out-of-Hospital Birth

C. Risk Screening for Appropriateness for Out-of-Hospital Birth

D. Transfer Plans/Back-up Physician and Hospital

E. Home Visits/Home Assessment

F. Supplies and Equipment

IX   Preconception Care

A. Risk Assessment

    1. Nutritional and weight considerations

        a. Folic acid and vitamin deficiencies

        b. Anemias

    2. Exposure/intake of potential teratogens

        a. Medications

        b. Vitamins

        c. Radiation

        d. Chemicals/Solvents/Pesticides

        e. Alcohol

        f. Tobacco

        g. Caffeine

        h. Drugs

        i. Heavy metals (lead and mercury)

        j. Infectious agents

    3. Medical Risk Factors

        a. Age

        b. Genetic diseases

        c. Diabetes

        d. Cardiovascular

        e. Hypertension

        f. Kidney disease

        g. Epilepsy

        h. Asthma

        i. Thyroid disease

        j. Cancer

        k. Lupus

        l. Infectious Diseases

        m. Psychiatric Illness

        n. Reproductive Health Tract Disorders

    4. Genetic Risk Factors

    5. Psychosocial Risk Factors

B. Diagnostic Tests

C. Intervention/Management/Patient Education

    1. Health promotion

    2. Folic acid and vitamin supplementation

    3. Immunizations

    4. Treatment of medical conditions

    5. Changes/elimination of medication regimes

    6. Genetic counseling

    7. Alcohol/Drug rehabilitation programs

8. Education on prevention of infectious diseases including STI's
9. Education on prevention of exposure to environmental/occupational hazards
10. Referrals as appropriate
11. Counseling/education as appropriate

Chapter 5 Questions

Care of the HIV-Infected Woman and Other Special Primary Care Circumstances

1. Which of the following BEST describes when preconception counseling should take place?
    a. 3 to 6 months before a pregnancy is planned
    b. 12 months before a pregnancy is planned
    c. When a woman requests it
    d. At every visit with a woman of childbearing age

2. An African-American client is at MOST risk for being a carrier of the gene that causes which of the following disorders?
    a. Cystic fibrosis
    b. Sickle-cell disease
    c. Canavan disease
    d. Tay-Sachs disease

3. Which of the following is NOT a responsibility of a midwife in the care of lesbian or bisexual women?
    a. To be aware of sexual practices among this population in order to counsel appropriately about safer sex measures
    b. To not make assumptions about the need or lack of need for contraceptive methods
    c. To encourage the woman to disclose to you her sexual preference so that you can most adequately target your teaching and management plan
    d. To use language either verbal or nonverbal that does not project a heterosexual bias

4. Which of the following substances is considered a central nervous system depressant?
    a. Marijuana
    b. Alcohol
    c. Cocaine
    d. Amphetamines

5. Which of the following situations BEST illustrates the phenomenon of "cross-tolerance"?
    a. When, due to chronic alcohol use, an individual needs more alcohol to produce the same effect than was needed before tolerance was developed
    b. When, due to chronic alcohol use, an individual needs less alcohol to produce the same effect than was needed as before tolerance was developed
    c. When an individual who has developed a tolerance to alcohol needs higher dosages of hypnotics to achieve an effect
    d. When an individual who has developed a tolerance to alcohol needs lower dosages of hypnotics to achieve an effect

■ **DATA FOR ITEM 6**

A woman who is an alcoholic asks you whether or not she should breastfeed. She has abused alcohol during pregnancy and has not expressed a commitment to cutting down or quitting her alcohol intake.

6. What is the BEST answer to this woman's question?
   a. It is generally believed that the benefits of breastmilk outweigh the risks of the infant ingesting any alcohol passed through the breastmilk.
   b. That breastfeeding is only recommended if she can cut down to 2–3 drinks per day
   c. That alcohol is not passed through breastmilk in large enough quantities to affect the infant so that breastfeeding is not contraindicated
   d. That the risks to the infant from any alcohol transmitted through breastmilk outweigh the benefits and that, therefore, breastfeeding is contraindicated for women who abuse alcohol

7. The human immunodeficiency virus (HIV) is which of the following types of viruses?
   a. Rhabdovirus
   b. Andenovirus
   c. Retrovirus
   d. Coxsackievirus

8. Which of the following cells that comprise the human immune system does the human immunodeficiency virus (HIV) target?
   a. B lymphocytes
   b. T4 lymphocytes
   c. T8 lymphocytes
   d. Macrophage

9. Which of the following statements BEST describes what is referred to as the "window phase" of human immunodeficiency virus (HIV) infection?
   a. The time between infection with HIV and the development of acquired immunodeficiency syndrome (AIDS)
   b. The time between infection with HIV and the development of the first symptoms of infection
   c. The time between infection with HIV and the development of detectable levels of antibodies in the plasma
   d. The time between infection with HIV and the development of HIV viremia

10. Globally, by which mode of transmission have MOST women become infected with the human immunodeficiency virus (HIV)?
   a. Vertical transmission
   b. Heterosexual transmission
   c. IV drug use
   d. Blood transfusions

11. Which of the following laboratory tests is most commonly used as the first test in the initial evaluation of HIV status?
   a. Enzyme-linked immunosorbent assay (ELISA)
   b. Western-blot
   c. Viral culture
   d. Polymerase chain reaction technique (PCR)

12. Which of the following laboratory tests is most likely to give a false-positive result for infection with HIV?
   a. Enzyme-linked immunosorbent assay (ELISA)
   b. Western-blot
   c. Viral culture
   d. Polymerase chain reaction technique (PCR)

13. What is the approximate risk of perinatal HIV transmission without antiretroviral treatment?

    a. 45%

    b. 40%

    c. 25%

    d. 20%

14. What is the approximate risk of perinatal HIV transmission with maternal zidovudine (ZDV) treatment during pregnancy and labor and ZDV treatment for the newborn?

    a. 20%

    b. 16%

    c. 12%

    d. 8%

15. Which of the following is the MOST common presenting clinical condition in women with HIV infection?

    a. Recurrent or recalcitrant condylomata acuminata

    b. Recurrent or recalcitrant *Candida* vaginitis

    c. Cervical neoplasia

    d. *Pneumocystis carinii* pneumonia

■ DATA FOR ITEM 16

During an initial physical examination on a woman who has just tested positive for HIV, a Mantoux test for tuberculosis infection was performed. Forty-eight hours later, the woman returns to have the results of the Mantoux test read. You note that there is not an induration on the arm where you injected the purified protein derivative (PPD).

16. What is the BEST interpretation and management of this result?

    a. The woman is not infected with tuberculosis, and no further testing or treatment is necessary.

    b. The woman could have been infected in the last 6 to 14 weeks or the test could be a false-negative, so a repeat Mantoux test should be performed in approximately 12 months.

    c. The negative test could be due to anergy, therefore, an anergy panel is indicated to verify the negative result.

    d. The negative test could be due to anergy, therefore a chest X-ray should be ordered.

17. Which of the following diseases needs to be managed and treated differently in a woman with HIV infection?

    a. Candidiasis

    b. Urinary tract infection (UTI)

    c. Gonorrhea or chlamydia

    d. Syphillis

18. Which of the following is the prophylactic treatment of choice against pnemocystis carinii pneumonia (PCP)?

    a. Metronidazole

    b. Penicillin G

    c. Bactrim (TMP-SMX)

    d. Rifabutin

19. Maternal HIV infection has NOT been associated with which of the following adverse fetal effects?

    a. Prematurity

    b. Stillbirth

    c. Intrauterine infection

    d. Congenital malformations

20. How soon after birth should an infant born to an HIV-infected woman start receiving zidovudine (ZDV)?

   a. Within 12 hours

   b. At 24 hours

   c. At 2 weeks

   d. At 2 months

DATA FOR ITEMS 21–22

You are caring for an HIV-infected woman who just gave birth to a term infant. The woman wants the infant tested to determine if the child is infected.

21. Which of the following tests should be administered to the newborn to determine its HIV status?

   a. Enzyme-linked immunosorbent assay (ELISA)

   b. Western-blot

   c. Viral culture and Polymerase chain reaction technique (PCR)

   d. Enzyme-linked immunosorbent assay (ELISA) and a CD4 count

ADDITIONAL DATA FOR ITEM 22

The results of the initial testing are positive.

22. What is the BEST interpretation and management of these results?

   a. Due to the high sensitivity of the testing conducted, the infant should be considered to be HIV-infected and his care managed accordingly.

   b. The positive test results indicate a high chance that the infant is infected, but you will be unable to tell for sure until testing at approximately 18 months of age when the infant can generate its own immune response.

   c. The positive test results indicate a high chance that the infant is infected, but to confirm the diagnosis, repeat testing using the same tests is indicated.

   d. The tests have a high false-positive result rate, therefore, confirmation of the results is indicated by conducting more specific testing.

Chapter 5 Answer Key

Care of the HIV-Infected Woman and Other Special Primary Care Situations

1. *d* p. 133

2. *b* p. 134

3. *c* p. 168–169

4. *b* p. 176

5. *c* p. 176

6. *d* p. 179

7. *c* p. 182

8. *b* p. 182

9. *c* p. 182

10. *b* p. 184

11. *a* p. 185

12. *a* p. 79 PM

13. *c* p. 187

14. *d* p. 187

15. *b* p. 189

16. *c* p. 191

17. *d* p. 192–193

18. *c* p. 193

19. *d* p. 193

20. *a* p. 196

21. *c* p. 196

22. *c* p. 196

55

PART III: ANTEPARTUM CARE

PART III

Chapter 6 Outline
The Normal Antepartum

I. Length of Human Gestation

    A. Gestational age by last menstrual period vs. gestational age by date of fertilization

II. Trimesters

    A. Length

    B. Milestones

III. Goals of Prenatal Care/Frequency of Prenatal Visits

IV. Fetal Growth and Development

    A. Developmental milestones (implantation, initiation of fetal heart activity, development of external genitalia, etc.)

    B. Embryonic vs. Fetal period

    C. Susceptibility to teratogens

V. Placental Growth and Development

    A. Anatomy and physiology of the placenta

    B. Function of the placenta

    C. Fetal circulation

VI. Diagnosis of Pregnancy

    A. Signs of pregnancy (presumptive, probable, positive)

    B. Pregnancy tests

        1. Types

        2. Timing

        3. Accuracy/Sensitivity

VII. Dating of a Pregnancy/Calculating Gestational Age/Estimated Date of Delivery

    A. Menstrual history

    B. Naegel's rule

    C. Fundal height

    D. Abdominal exam/Leopold's maneuvers

    E. Uterine sizing

    F. Fetal heart tones

G. Quickening

H. Ultrasound examination

VIII. Determination/Notation of Gravity and Parity

IX. Initial Visit

A. Components of the medical, surgical, social, family, obstetrical, gynecologic, nutritional, and menstrual histories

B. Components of the history of the current pregnancy

C. Components of the initial antepartal physical and pelvic examination

D. Routine laboratory test and adjunctive studies for the initial antepartal visit

(See Table 1 at the end of this section for "Routine Prenatal Laboratory Tests and Adjunctive Studies")

1. Purpose

2. Indications

3. Timing

4. Interpretation

5. Management

E. Additional/Non-routine testing

(See Table 2 at the end of this section for "Additional/Non-routine Prenatal Laboratory Tests and Adjunctive Studies")

1. Purpose

2. Indications

3. Timing

4. Interpretation

5. Management

X. Revisits

A. Components of chart review/interval history

B. Components of interval physical exam

C. Laboratory tests and adjunctive studies (diabetes screen, repeats of VDRL, cultures, hematocrit/hemoglobin, antibody screen, GBS screen, etc.)

1. Purpose of each test

2. Indications for each test

3. Timing for each test

4. Interpretation of test results

5. Management of test results

XI. Maternal Anatomical and Physiological Changes/Discomforts of Pregnancy

(See Table 3 at the end of this section for "Common Discomforts of Pregnancy")

A. Physiological cause for discomforts/Usual timing in pregnancy

B. Anticipatory Guidance

C. Relief measures

D. Differentiation of normal physiological changes from symptoms of pathologic process

XII. Maternal Psychological Adjustment

XIII. Additional Components of Antepartal Teaching

A. Nutrition and exercise in pregnancy (Discussed in more detail in Chapter 8)

B. Substance abuse during pregnancy

C. Medications during pregnancy
FDA Pregnancy Risk Categories for Drugs

D. Immunizations during pregnancy

E. Household/Occupational hazards

F. Screening for domestic violence

G. Travel in pregnancy

H. Work during pregnancy

XIV. Screening for Maternal and Fetal Complications (Addressed further in Chapters 9 and 10)

■ **Table 1 Routine/Initial Antepartal Laboratory Studies**

- Pap smear
- Gonococcal (GC) and chlamydial (CT) culture
- Blood type
- Rh factor
- Antibody screen
- Sickledex (sickle cell prep) or hemoglobin electrophoresis
- Tuberculin test (PPD)
- Serologic testing for syphilis (VDRL, RPR, etc.)
- Hepatitis B surface antigen (HbSAg)
- Rubella titer
- Varicella antibody screen
- Hemoglobin and Hematocrit/CBC
- Urinalysis/Urine culture

■ **Table 2 Additional Laboratory Studies for Particular Gestational Age, Revisits, or Specific Maternal Risks**

- Diabetes screen
- Maternal serum alphafetoprotein (AFP)/Triple Screen
- HIV antibody test
- Group B streptococcus culture (Know GBS Protocols)
- Repeat serologic testing for syphilis
- Repeat Hematocrit/Hemoglobin
- Repeat antibody screen
- Repeat GC/Chlamydia
- Urine dipstick tests

■ **Table 3 Common Discomforts of Pregnancy**

- Backache
- Bleeding and swelling of gums
- Breast tenderness/Breast leakage/Changes in breast size
- Changes in libido
- Constipation
- Dependent edema
- Dizziness/Faintness/Supine Hypotensive Syndrome
- Dyspareunia
- Fatigue
- Flatulence
- Headaches
- Heartburn
- Hemorrhoids
- Hyperventilation/Shortness of breath
- Leg cramps
- Leukorrhea
- Nasal congestion/Nosebleeds
- Nausea/Vomiting
- Ptyalism
- Round ligament pain
- Sciatica
- Skin changes (chloasma, discolorations, stretch marks)
- Tingling and Numbness of Fingers
- Urinary frequency
- Varicosities

Chapter 6 Questions
The Normal Antepartum

1. What is the length, from the day of fertilization, of human gestation?
   a. 294 days
   b. 280 days
   c. 266 days
   d. 252 days

2. Which of the following is responsible for maintaining the corpus luteum of pregnancy?
   a. Progesterone
   b. Human placental lactogen (HPL)
   c. Human chorionic gonadotropin (hCG)
   d. Alpha-fetoprotein (AFP)

■   DATA FOR ITEM 3

A client calls to inform you that she is five days overdue for her menstrual period. She says that she took a home pregnancy test and that the results were negative. She asks you what she should do.

3. Which of the following is the MOST accurate response to this question?
   a. Home pregnancy tests are very accurate, so if the test was negative she probably is not pregnant and should wait for her period to arrive.
   b. Home pregnancy tests are very accurate, but that she should wait a few days and then repeat the urine pregnancy test either at home or at the clinic.
   c. Home pregnancy tests are inaccurate, so she should come to your office for a clinical urine test, which is more accurate.
   d. Home pregnancy tests are unreliable and should be followed by a blood pregnancy test at the clinic to confirm the results.

4. Which of the following anatomical or physiological changes of pregnancy is thought to be caused by estrogen?
   a. Hypertrophy of the uterine wall
   b. Increase in maternal basal body temperature
   c. Excessive salivation
   d. Relaxation of the vascular walls

5. In terms of the maternal psychological processes of pregnancy, the first trimester of pregnancy is often described as which of the following?
   a. The period of radiant health
   b. The period of watchful waiting
   c. The period of adjustment
   d. The period of maternal role resolution

6. The fusion of the pronuclei of the sperm and ovum that happens with fertilization produces which of the following?
   a. The embryo
   b. The zygote
   c. The morula
   d. The blastocyst

7. Implantation begins approximately how soon after fertilization?

    a. 2 days

    b. 6 days

    c. 10 days

    d. 14 days

8. Which of the following is TRUE regarding the embryonic period?

    a. It starts at fertilization and continues through day 48 of fetal development.

    b. It starts at the end of implantation and continues through day 48 of fetal development.

    c. It starts at fertilization and continues through day 56 of fetal development.

    d. It starts approximately 7 days after fertilization and proceeds through day 56 of fetal development.

9. The eyelids of a fetus remain fused through what gestational age by LMP?

    a. 15th week

    b. 20th week

    c. 25th week

    d. 30th week

10. Which of the following is TRUE regarding the first two weeks of gestation?

    a. The embryo is particularly susceptible to the effects of teratogens

    b. Primitive placental circulation is established

    c. The three main germ layers of the embryo develop

    d. The primitive cardiovascular system and blood cells develop

11. Which of the following is the definition of the decidua?

    a. The uterine endometrium during a woman's reproductive years

    b. The uterine endometrium during pregnancy

    c. The part of the uterine endometrium where implantation occurs

    d. The part of the uterine endometrium that is not shed immediately post-partum

12. Which of the following is the function of the umbilical arteries?

    a. To carry oxygenated blood to the fetus

    b. To carry oxygenated blood to the placenta

    c. To carry poorly oxygenated blood to the placenta

    d. To carry poorly oxygenated blood to the fetus

13. Which of the following is NOT a function of the placenta?

    a. Exchange of oxygen-carbon dioxide

    b. Synthesis of cholesterol and fatty acids

    c. Transfer of maternal antibodies

    d. Filtering of infectious organisms

HD, a 26-year-old G1P0, comes to see you for her initial prenatal visit at 10 weeks gestational age by LMP and confirmed by ultrasound. When you ask her about medication use she states that she had a migraine headache during the week before her period was due for which she first took some aspirin and then took a narcotic analgesic prescribed to her by her primary physician. She also states that until two weeks ago she had been taking oral tetracycline and using topical Retin-A cream for acne.

14. In terms of potential teratogenic effects to the fetus, you are MOST concerned by the use of which of the following?

   a. The aspirin
   b. The narcotic analgesic
   c. The tetracycline
   d. The Retin-A cream

LT is a 24-year-old G0P0 who comes to see you on 8/24/00. Her last menstrual period was six weeks ago on 7/13/00. She states that in the last three weeks she has had intermittent nausea with some occasional vomiting. She also complains of breast tenderness and fatigue. Upon physical examination you note that her breasts have some nodularity and tenseness and that her vaginal mucosa and cervix have a bluish tint.

15. LT has which of the following signs of pregnancy?

   a. Probable
   b. Presumptive
   c. Possible
   d. Positive

16. Which of the following is TRUE regarding the blue tint of LT's cervix?

   a. It is referred to as Chadwick's sign and is a result of increased hemoglobin in maternal circulation.
   b. It is referred to as Chadwick's sign and is the result of increased vascularity and vasocongestion.
   c. It is referred to as Hegar's sign and is the result of increased hemoglobin in maternal circulation.
   d. It is referred to as Hegar's sign and is the result of increased vascularity and vasogongestion.

17. You perform a pregnancy test using a urine sample and it comes back positive. Using Naegele's rule, which of the following is LT's estimated date of delivery (EDD)?

   a. 4/20/01
   b. 12/16/01
   c. 5/20/01
   d. 4/16/01

18. Based on LT's EGA by LMP, which of the following is MOST appropriate to include as a part of your anticipatory guidance during this visit?

   a. Relief measures for round ligament pain
   b. Relief measures for heartburn
   c. Relief measures for tingling and numbness of the fingers
   d. Relief measures for nocturia

■ **DATA FOR ITEMS 19–20**

MS is a 32-year-old who is currently pregnant and has had four previous pregnancies. Her abbreviated obstetrical history is as follows: she has had one first trimester induced abortion and one spontaneous abortion at 10 weeks gestational age; she has also had one premature live birth and a full-term delivery of twins. The twins are currently alive and well, but the infant who was born prematurely died during the first week following its birth.

19. Using the two-digit system to designate gravity and parity, which of the following is accurate to describe MS?
   a. G5P1
   b. G5P2
   c. G5P3
   d. G5P4

20. Using a four-digit system to designate gravity and parity, which of the following is accurate to describe MS?
   a. G5P2222
   b. G5P1121
   c. G5P1122
   d. G5P2122

21. For a woman at 13 weeks gestational age who is coming for her first prenatal appointment, all of the following are routine laboratory exams except:
   a. Blood type
   b. Hepatitis B surface antigen test
   c. Maternal serum alpha–fetoprotein
   d. Serology test for syphilis

22. Which of the following is NOT routinely used by midwives to monitor fetal growth?
   a. Fundal height
   b. Ultrasound
   c. Estimated fetal weight
   d. Abdominal palpation

■ **DATA FOR ITEM 23**

TL is a 16-year-old G1P0 at 10 weeks gestational age by LMP who is seeing you for her initial prenatal physical exam. She has no complaints and her vital signs are all within normal limits. Her routine prenatal laboratory work, which was obtained during her orientation visit, is all within normal limits as well. Her physical exam is unremarkable except that as you prepare to perform the pelvic examination, she becomes agitated, starts to cry, and refuses the exam.

23. Which of the following is the BEST course of action at this time?
   a. Let her know that it is common to be afraid, help her to relax with breathing exercises, assure her that you will be gentle, and try again to perform the exam.
   b. Help her to calm down, explain to her that it is important to her health and to the health of her baby that you get the information from the pelvic exam as early in pregnancy as possible, and reschedule the exam for later that week.
   c. Explore with her the reasons for her refusal, explain why you need to perform the exam, and if necessary, postpone the exam for later in pregnancy.
   d. Get someone else in the office who is more persuasive or experienced in dealing with young women to either help you perform the exam or to do the exam for you.

24. Which of the following is an appropriate recommendation for relief of pregnancy-induced leukorrhea?
  a. Warm sitz baths followed by thorough drying of the entire genital area
  b. Warm sterile water douches
  c. Corn starch applied to a sanitary napkin
  d. Frequent changes of cotton-crotch panties

25. All of the following are causes of nonpathological urinary frequency during pregnancy EXCEPT which of the following?
  a. Decreased room for distention of the bladder
  b. Sporadic, progesterone-induced spasm of the bladder
  c. Anteflexion of the enlarging uterus
  d. Pressure of the fetal presenting part

DATA FOR ITEM 26

FS comes to see you for a routine prenatal appointment at 32 weeks. She states that she has been feeling short of breath lately. After confirming that there is no likely pathological cause for the shortness of breath, you inform her that shortness of breath is a common complaint of women at this point in pregnancy. You know that this pregnancy-induced shortness of breath is due in part to the enlarging fetus and uterus.

26. Which of the following is another non-pathological cause of shortness of breath of pregnancy?
  a. Descent of the diaphragm
  b. Increased carbon dioxide levels
  c. Increase in the functional residual volume of air in the lungs
  d. Widening of the transverse diameter of the thoracic cage

27. Which of the following is NOT used as a means of dating a pregnancy?
  a. Quantitative serum hCG
  b. "Sure" date for LMP
  c. Uterine sizing
  d. Ultrasound

DATA FOR ITEM 28

A pregnant client has been taking diazepam as an anxiolytic. When you look this medication up in a drug reference manual to determine potential risk to the fetus, you read that "there is positive evidence of human fetal risk, but the benefits from use in pregnant women may be acceptable despite the risk."

28. This description corresponds to which of the FDA Pregnancy Risk Categories for Drugs?
  a. Category X
  b. Category B
  c. Category C
  d. Category D

29. Which of the following is TRUE regarding immunization of women in pregnancy?
  a. The risk to the fetus of a live-virus vaccine is reduced during the last part of the second trimester through birth.
  b. Immunization with varicella immune globulin can be considered in exposed pregnant women.
  c. Immunization against rubella is recommended in third trimester for exposed pregnant women.
  d. The risk to the fetus from tetanus-diphtheria inactivated bacterial vaccines outweighs the risk of maternal tetanus, so immunization in an exposed pregnant women should be avoided.

30. Which of the following components of an abdominal examination of a pregnant woman would be MOST useful in helping to confirm the estimated gestational age of a pregnancy at approximately 9 weeks gestational age?
  a. Observation for linea nigra
  b. Fundal height
  c. Checking for fetal heart tones with doppler
  d. Uterine sizing

31. Which of the following is TRUE regarding serum B-hCG in a normal pregnancy?
  a. It can be detected within 9 to 11 days following conception.
  b. It peaks at 20 weeks gestation.
  c. It doubles every 24 hours in the first weeks of pregnancy.
  d. It returns to nearly non-pregnant levels during the third trimester.

Chapter 6 Answer Key
The Normal Antepartum

1. *c* p. 229

2. *c* p. 229

3. *b* p. 232

4. *a* p. 232

5. *c* p. 235

6. *b* p. 238

7. *b* p. 238–239

8. *b* p. 238–239

9. *c* p. 243

10. *b* p. 239

11. *b* p. 244

12. *c* p. 245–246

13. *d* p. 247

14. *c* p. 278

15. *b* p. 251

16. *b* p. 232

17. *a* p. 255

18. *d* p. 270

19. *b* p. 254

20. *d* p. 254

21. *c* p. 259

22. *b* p. 260

23. *c* p. 258

24. *d* p. 267

25. *b* p. 267

26. *b* p. 272

27. *a* p. 257–258

28. *d* p. 278

29. *b* p. 281

30. *d* p. 233–234

31. *a* p. 284

Chapter 7 Outline

Obstetrical Abdominal Exam and Clinical Pelvimetry

I. **Obstetrical Abdominal Exam**

   A. Measuring fundal height

   Technique

       a. Palpation/Comparison to expected fundal height for gestational age

       b. Calipers

       c. Tape measure

       i. Following abdominal contour

ii) **Without abdominal contour**

   B. Abdominal palpation

      1. Uterine tone, tenderness, consistency, contractility

      2. Abdominal muscle tone

      3. Detection fetal movement

      4. Estimation of fetal weight

      5. Determination of fetal lie, presentation, position, and variety

      6. Determination of engagement of fetal presenting part

   C. Leopold's Maneuvers

      1. First maneuver

      2. Second maneuver

      3. Third maneuver (Pawlik's maneuver/Pawlik's grip)

      4. Fourth maneuver

   D. Location of fetal heart tones (FHT's)

   E. Assessment of diastasis

II. **Clinical Pelvimetry**

   A. Pelvic anatomy

      1. Pelvic bones/structures

      2. Pelvic planes

      3. Pelvic diameters

    B. Pelvic types (Caldwell-Moloy Classification)
        1. Gynecoid
        2. Android
        3. Anthropoid
        4. Platypelloid

    Know the following for each of the above pelvic types:
        a. Distinguishing characteristics
        b. Potential effects on labor and birth

    C. Clinical pelvimetry
        1. Technique
        2. Parameters of normal
        3. Deviations from normal
        4. Evaluation of findings/Determining pelvic adequacy

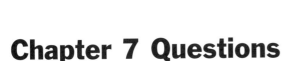

Chapter 7 Questions

Obstetrical Abdominal Exam and Clinical Pelvimetry

1. Which of the following will be MOST helpful in ensuring accurate monitoring of fetal growth using fundal height?
   a. Using calipers
   b. Having the same examiner perform the measurements
   c. Having a second person confirm the measurements
   d. Using the same tape measurer

DATA FOR ITEM 2

You are performing an abdominal exam on a woman at approximately 16 weeks gestational age.

2. Where would you expect to feel her uterine fundus?
   a. Two fingerbreadths above the symphysis pubis
   b. Halfway between the symphysis pubis and umbilicus
   c. One to two fingerbreadths below the umbilicus
   d. At the umbilicus

3. Measurement of abdominal girth in a woman of average size is a helpful adjunct to fundal height in the diagnosis of which of the following conditions?
   a. Polyhydramnios
   b. Trophoblastic disease
   c. Macrosomia
   d. Abnormal lie

4. Which of the following part of the hands should be used for abdominal examination?
   a. Fingertips
   b. Palmar surface of fingers
   c. Palms of the hands
   d. Heels of the hands

DATA FOR ITEM 5

As you observe the contour of a woman's uterus, you note that there is a saucer-like depression just below the umbilicus and a bulge like a full bladder above the symphysis pubis.

5. This is indicative of which of the following?
   a. A transverse lie
   b. A breech presentation
   c. An anterior position
   d. A posterior position

6. In a face presentation, which of the following will be the cephalic prominence that is palpable during the fourth Leopold's maneuver?
   a. The occiput
   b. The sinciput
   c. The bregma
   d. The mentum

7. Which of the following is the cephalic prominence that is palpable during the fourth Leopold's maneuver in a well-flexed cephalic presentation?

a. The occiput
b. The sinciput
c. The bregma
d. The mentum

■ **DATA FOR ITEM 8**

During an abdominal examination of a woman at term you feel the cephalic prominence on the same side as the fetal parts.

8. This is indicative of which of the following?

a. Face presentation
b. Vertex presentation
c. Brow presentation
d. Sinciput(Military) presentation

■ **DATA FOR ITEM 9**

During an abdominal examination of a woman at term both your hands simultaneously encounter a hard mass that is equally prominent on both sides.

9. This is indicative of which of the following?

a. Face presentation
b. Vertex presentation
c. Brow presentation
d. Sinciput (Military) presentation

10. The pelvis is comprised of how many bones?

a. Three
b. Four
c. Five
d. Six

11. Which of the following demarcations divides the false and the true pelvis?

a. The sacroiliac synchondrosis
b. The sacroiliac notch
c. The linea terminalis
d. The ischial spine

12. Which of the following is the smallest pelvic diameter to which the fetus has to accommodate itself?

a. The obstetrical conjugate
b. The conjugata vera
c. The interspinous diameter
d. The intertuberous diameter

13. Which of the following is the only diameter of the pelvic inlet that can be measured clinically?

a. The diagonal conjugate
b. The obstetrical conjugate
c. The conjugata vera
d. The oblique diameter

14. Which of the following planes of the pelvis is known as the "plane of least dimensions?"

   a. The inlet

   b. The midplane

   c. The outlet

15. Which is the minimal measurement of the angle of the pubic arch that determines adequacy of the pelvic outlet?

   a. 45°

   b. 80°

   c. 90°

   d. 120°

◼ DATA FOR ITEM 16

The following are the findings of clinical pelvimetry performed on JH, a 24-year-old G2P0010:

Inlet—oval with forepelvis more narrow than posterior pelvis; anteroposterior diameter much larger than transverse diameter

Sacrum—the sacrum is flat, long, and posteriorly inclined

Sacrosciatic notch—wide

Sidewalls—somewhat convergent

Ischial spines—prominent but not encroaching

Pubic arch—slightly narrow

16. Based on this information, which of the following BEST describes JH's type of pelvis?

   a. Android

   b. Anthropoid

   c. Gynecoid

   d. Platypelloid

17. Which of the following is the LEAST common type of pelvis among women?

   a. Android

   b. Anthropoid

   c. Gynecoid

   d. Platypelloid

18. Anthropoid pelvises are MOST associated with which of the following?

   a. Fetopelvic disproportion

   b. Deep transverse arrest of labor

   c. Posterior position of the fetus

   d. Shoulder dystocia

19. Which of the following is the shortest anteroposterior diameter of the pelvis?

   a. The conjugata vera

   b. The obstetrical conjugate

   c. The diagonal conjugate

   d. The anteroposterior diameter of the plane of least dimensions

20. What is the BEST way to test adequacy of the pelvis?

   a. Clinical pelvimetry

   b. Trial of labor

   c. X-ray evaluation of pelvis

   d. Ultrasound evaluation of pelvis and fetus

Chapter 7 Answer Key
Obstetrical Abdominal Exam and Clinical Pelvimetry

1. *b* p. 731

2. *b* p. 732

3. *a* p. 733

4. *b* p. 734

5. *d* p. 737

6. *a* p. 739

7. *b* p. 739

8. *b* p. 739

9. *d* p. 739

10. *b* p. 791

11. *c* p. 791

12. *c* p. 794

13. *a* p. 793

14. *b* p. 794

15. *c* p. 795

16. *b* p. 797

17. *d* p. 797

18. *c* p. 796

19. *b* p. 793

20. *b* p. 484

Chapter 8 Outline
Nutrition and Exercise in Pregnancy

I.   Fetal Effects of Maternal Nutritional Status/Intake

    A. Fetal birth weight

      1. Parameters of Normal

      2. Interrelationship with maternal nutritional status

      3. Interrelationship with gestational age

    B. Fetal growth and development

      1. Cell hyperplasia vs. cell hypertrophy

      2. Symmetrical vs. asymmetrical growth retardation

      3. Appropriate size for gestational age (AGA)

      4. Small for gestational age (SGA)

      5. Large for gestational age (LGA)

    Know the following for each of the above terms:

      a. Definition

      b. Interrelationship with maternal nutrition

      c. Appropriate interventions for deviations from normal

II.   Assessment of Maternal Weight Gain in Pregnancy

    A. Components of weight gain in pregnancy

    B. Recommended total weight gain parameters

    C. Recommended weight gain by trimesters

    D. Body Mass Index (BMI) calculations

III. Undernutrition/Underweight/Nutritional Stress/Overweight

    A. Definition

    B. Necessary nutritional interventions

IV.   Nutritional Needs During Pregnancy

    A. Caloric needs

    B. Protein needs

    C. Mineral needs

      1. Iron

      2. Calcium

      3. Zinc

      4. Magnesium

    D. Vitamin needs

      1. Vitamin A

      2. Vitamin C

3. Vitamin D

4. Vitamin E

5. Vitamin B_6

6. Folate/Folic acid

E. Fluid needs

Know the following for each of the above

1. The Recommended Daily Dietary Allowances (RDA) for pregnancy

2. Food sources

V.   Nutritional Assessment

A. Anthropometric measures

1. Pre-pregnancy Weight/Height/BMI

2. Weight gain in pregnancy

B. Lab/Diagnostic tests

1. Hematocrit/Hemoglobin

2. Serum iron/Total iron-binding capacity (TIBC)

3. Red blood cell count

4. Serum ferritin/transferrin

5. Glucose screen

6. Urinalysis (protein/glucose dipstick)

C. Nutritional/Dietary History or Recall

The Food Pyramid/Recommended daily servings of food groups

VI.   Nutritional Interventions

A. Patient education/counseling

1. Diet modifications

2. Physical activity/Exercise

B. Vitamin/Mineral supplementation

C. Referral to dietitian/Medical nutrition therapy

D. Referral to WIC/Food assistance programs

VII.   Nutritional High Risk Populations

A. Tobacco use/Substance abuse

B. Lactose intolerance

C. Multiple gestation

D. Strict vegetarianism

E. Food allergies

F. Teenagers

G. Hyperemesis gravidarium/Pernicious vomiting

H. Short interconceptional period

I. Poor obstetrical history

J. Failure to gain 10 lbs. by 20 weeks pregnancy

K. Serious emotional upset/problems

L. Anorexia nervosa/Bulimia/Binge-eating

M. Pica

N. Gestational diabetes mellitus (GDM)

Know the following for each of the above conditions:
1. Definition
2. Effects on nutritional status
3. Necessary nutritional interventions

VIII. Maternal Effects of Exercise During Pregnancy

A. Cardiovascular and hemodynamics

B. Thermoregulation

C. Metabolism

D. Respiration/Acid-base balance

E. Biomechanics

F. Psychological

IX. Fetal Effects of Exercise

A. Uterine blood flow

B. Thermoregulation

C. Fetal cardiovascular response

X. Management of Exercise in Pregnancy

A. Baseline database
1. Current level of activity/physical condition
2. Weight/nutritional status
3. Interest/motivation to exercise

B. Screening
1. Obstetrical/Medical contraindications to exercise
2. Obstetrical/Medical conditions that may benefit from exercise

C. Developing exercise prescription
1. Goals of exercise
2. Appropriate type(s) and intensity of exercise
3. Special exercises for pregnancy
4. Safety considerations
5. Biomechanics
6. Monitoring criteria
   a. Heart rate
   b. Hydration
   c. Temperature

        d. Caloric expenditure

        e. Warning signs that indicate need for immediate cessation of exercise

        f. Fatigue

    D. Monitoring/Assessment

      1. Warning signs

      2. Weight trends/Fundal height/Fetal growth

      3. Adjustments to exercise regime as indicated

      4. Attainment of goals

Chapter 8 Questions

Nutrition and Exercise in Pregnancy

■ **DATA FOR ITEM 1**

TR is an 18-year-old G1P0 at 39 weeks gestational age. She is 5'3" tall and now weighs 138 lb. Her pre-pregnancy weight was 115 lb.

1. How would you categorize TR's total pregnancy weight gain?

   a. Insufficient

   b. Adequate

   c. Excessive

   d. Average

2. Which of the following is LEAST likely to affect a newborn's birth weight?

   a. Maternal parity

   b. Maternal pre-pregnancy weight

   c. Maternal height

   d. Gestational age

3. Which of the following terms is used to describe an increase in the number of cells by cell division?

   a. Hypertrophy

   b. Hyperplasia

   c. Hypermeiosis

   d. Hypermitosis

■ **DATA FOR ITEMS 4–5**

Examination of a term newborn male reveals that the infant has suffered from significant intrauterine growth retardation/restriction (IUGR). His weight and abdominal circumference are below normal for gestational age, but his head circumference is within normal limits.

4. This newborn has suffered from which of the following?

   a. Symmetrical growth retardation

   b. Asymmetrical growth retardation

   c. Hypoplastic growth retardation

   d. Hypocaloric growth retardation

5. It is MOST likely that this infant's growth retardation (IUGR) was due to which of the following?

   a. Uteroplacental insufficiency

   b. Maternal caloric insufficiency

   c. Maternal protein deficiency

   d. Inadequate maternal weight gain during pregnancy

6. If the fetus suffers from malnutrition during the time of development when cells are increasing in size, then the damage suffered by the fetus is BEST characterized as which of the following?

   a. Irreversible

   b. Reversible

   c. Asymmetric

   d. Catabolic

7. Which of the following is the optimal birth weight range as demonstrated by studies on birth weight and perinatal morbidity and mortality?
   a. 2500 to 2999 grams
   b. 3000 to 3499 grams
   c. 3500 to 3999 grams
   d. 4000 to 4499 grams

8. What is the recommended daily dietary allowances (RDA) for calories and protein for pregnant women?
   a. 2200 calories and 50 grams of protein
   b. 2500 calories and 60 grams of protein
   c. 2500 calories and 50 grams of protein
   d. 2200 calories and 60 grams of protein

9. What is the recommended intake of folic acid during pregnancy?
   a. 1.0 mg
   b. 0.1 mg
   c. 0.4 mg
   d. 0.04 mg

10. What is the recommended daily dietary allowance (RDA) for calcium during pregnancy?
   a. 800 mg
   b. 1000 mg
   c. 1200 mg
   d. 1500 mg

11. What is the appropriate amount of Vitamin C supplementation during pregnancy?
   a. 150 mg
   b. 250 mg
   c. 350 mg
   d. 500 mg

12. Which of the following is considered a source of complete protein?
   a. Tofu
   b. Green peas
   c. Peanut butter
   d. Lentils

13. At what week gestational age is it important to re-evaluate a client's nutrition to ensure adequate diet during the peak in cellular growth of the fetal brain?
   a. 20 weeks
   b. 24 weeks
   c. 28 weeks
   d. 30 weeks

14. The Higgins Intervention Methodology for determining weight requirements uses which of the following to determine calorie and protein intake?
   a. Ideal body weight and individual activity level
   b. Ideal body weight and age
   c. Body-mass index (BMI) and age
   d. Body-mass index (BMI) and individual activity level

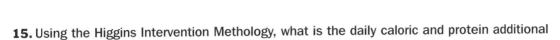
15. Using the Higgins Intervention Methology, what is the daily caloric and protein additional allowance at 20 weeks gestation?

   a. Adding 500 calories and 25 g of protein to the woman's nonpregnant requirements

   b. Adding 500 calories and 25 g of protein to the woman's first trimester requirements

   c. Adding 300 calories and 15 g of protein to the woman's first trimester requirements

   d. Adding 300 calories and 15 g of protein to the woman's nonpregnant requirements

■ **DATA FOR ITEM 16**

The following is GF's 24-hour recall diet history:

Breakfast:	Cold cereal
	Glass of orange juice
	Coffee
Mid-morning snack:	Glass of lemonade
	One banana
Lunch:	Glass of non-caffeinated soda
	Turkey breast sandwich with lettuce and cheese
	Cup of pasta salad
Mid-afternoon snack	Glass of water
	Saltine crackers with peanut butter
	Cup of grapes
Dinner	Glass of milk
	Vegetable and meat lasagna
	Frozen yogurt

16. GH needs to increase her intake of which of the following?

   a. Fruits and vegetables

   b. Fruits and breads/cereals/pastas

   c. Meat and vegetable

   d. Vegetables and breads/cereals/pastas

17. Which of the following has the highest iron content?

   a. Beef liver

   b. Soy beans

   c. Spinach

   d. Roast beef

18. Which of the following comprises the majority of dietary iron?

   a. Heme iron

   b. Nonheme iron

   c. Ferrous gluconate

   d. Ferrous sulfate

19. Which of the following is the BEST suggestion to increase the absorption of iron supplements?

   a. Take the supplement with a meal

   b. Take the supplement with milk

   c. Take the supplement with orange juice

   d. Take the supplement at the same time as prenatal vitamins

20. Exercise increases all of the following EXCEPT:

   a. Blood volume

   b. Vasculature

   c. Vascular resistance

   d. Cardiac output

21. Which of the following is considered to contribute to hypotensive syndrome in pregnancy?
  a. Increase in blood volume
  b. Increased relaxation of vasculature
  c. Increased heart rate
  d. Increase in hemoglobin concentration

22. Which of the following is TRUE regarding normal fetal cardiovascular response to exercise?
  a. The fetal heart rate decelerates during exercise in response to decreased uteroplacental blood flow.
  b. The fetal heart rate decelerates during exercise in response to decreased maternal blood oxygenation.
  c. The fetal heart accelerates during and after exercise in response to maternal exertion.
  d. The fetal heart rate remains the same during exercise due to fetal and placental adaptive mechanisms.

23. Which of the following is TRUE regarding the birth weight of infants born to women who exercised through most of pregnancy and then reduced or ceased exercise during the final months of pregnancy?
  a. They tend to have reduced birth weight due to low body-fat.
  b. They tend to have reduced birth weight due to smaller structure (small-for-gestational-age).
  c. They tend to have increased birth weight due to highly efficient placental function.
  d. They tend to have increased birth weight due to increased muscle mass.

24. For which of the following conditions in pregnancy is exercise an absolute contraindication?
  a. History of IUGR
  b. Multiple gestation
  c. Mitral valve prolapse
  d. Presence of an infection/fever

25. Which of the following activities should women avoid entirely throughout pregnancy?
  a. Cycling
  b. Ice-skating
  c. Downhill skiing
  d. Basketball

Chapter 8 Answer Key
Nutrition and Exercise in Pregnancy

1. *a* p. 321

2. *c* p. 317

3. *b* p. 318

4. *b* p. 318

5. *a* p. 318

6. *b* p. 318

7. *c* p. 318

8. *b* p. 319

9. *c* p. 134 PM

10. *c* p. 135 PM

11. *b* p. 320

12. *d* p. 138 PM

13. *c* p. 325

14. *a* p. 321

15. *a* p. 324

16. *d* p. 139 PM

17. *b* p. 133 PM

18. *b* p. 320

19. *c* p. 320

20. *c* p. 142

21. *b* p. 143

22. *c* p. 143–144

23. *c* p. 144

24. *d* p. 153

25. *c* p. 158–159

Chapter 9 Outline
Fetal Assessment

I.   Screening Tests vs. Diagnostic Tests

II.   Confirmation of Pregnancy/Assessment of Viability

  A. Signs/Symptoms of pregnancy (Discussed further in Chapter 6)

  B. Pregnancy tests
  • Quantitative vs. qualitative B-hCG tests

  C. Ultrasound examination

III. Alpha-Fetoprotein (AFP) Testing/Triple Marker Testing

  A. Definition

  B. Indications/Contraindications

  C. Technique/Timing

  D. Interpretation/Management of results

IV.   Genetic Counseling

  A. Indications (See Table 1 at the end of this section for "Indications for Genetic/High Risk Counseling and Genetic Testing)

  B. History taking

  C. Genetic screening tests

  D. Interpretation/management of results

V.   Chorionic Villus Sampling

  A. Definition

  B. Indications/Contraindications

  C. Risks

  D. Technique/Timing

  E. Interpretation/Management of results

VI.   Amniocentesis

  A. Definition

  B. Indications/Contraindications

  C. Risks

  D. Technique/Timing

  E. Interpretation/Management of results

VII.   Cordocentesis

    A. Definition

    B. Indications/Contraindications

    C. Risks

    D. Technique/Timing

    E. Interpretation/Management of results

VIII.   Fetal Movement Counts (FMC)

    A. Definition

    B. Indications

    C. Technique

    D. Interpretation/Management of results

IX.   Auscultated Acceleration Tests (AAT)

    A. Definition

    B. Indications

    C. Technique/Timing

    D. Interpretation/Management of results

X.   Nonstress Test (NST)

    A. Definition

    B. Indications

    C. Technique/Timing

    D. Interpretation/Management of results

XI.   Contraction Stress Test (CST)

    A. Definition

    B. Indications/Contraindications

    C. Risks

    D. Technique/Timing

    E. Interpretation/Management of results

XII.   Vibroacoustic Stimulation (VAS)

    A. Definition

    B. Indications/Contraindications

    C. Technique

    D. Interpretation/Management of results

XIII. Biophysical Profile

A. Definition

B. Indications

C. Technique/Criteria/Timing

D. Interpretation/Management of results

XIV. Modified Biophysical Profile

A. Definition

B. Indications

C. Technique/Criteria/Timing

D. Interpretation/Management of results

XV. Amniotic Fluid Index (AFI)

A. Definition

B. Indications

C. Technique

D. Interpretation/Management of results

XVI. Doppler Velocimetry

A. Definition

B. Indications

C. Technique

D. Interpretation/Management of results

XVII. Ultrasound

A. Definition

B. Indications

C. Technique/Criteria/Timing

D. Interpretation/Management of results

■   **Table 1 Indications for Genetic/High Risk Counseling or Genetic Testing**

- Advanced Maternal Age (AMA)
- Previous child with genetic abnormalities
- Family/Personal history of birth defects/mental retardation
- Congenital heart disease
- Neural tube defects
- Cleft lip/Cleft palate
- Multiple congenital anomalies
- Mental retardation
- Down syndrome
- Fragile X syndrome

- Family/Personal history of known/suspected Mendelian genetic disorder(s)
    - Cystic fibrosis
    - Hemophilia A or B
    - Duchenne muscular dystrophy
    - Becker muscular dystrophy
- Ethnicity
    - African
        - Sickle cell trait/Sickle cell disease
        - Thalessemias
    - Mediterranean/Middle Eastern/Asian
        - Thalessemias
    - Jewish
        - Tay-Sachs disease
        - Canavan disease
- Exposure to Teratogens
    - Medications/Drugs
        - Alcohol
        - Amnioglycosides
        - Angiotensin-coverting enzyme inhibitors (ACE Inhibitors)
        - Anticonvulsants
        - Antithyroid agents
        - Cocaine
        - Coumarin derivatives
        - Folic acid antagonists
        - Hormonal agents
        - Lithium salts
        - Retinoids/arotinoids
        - Tetracyclines
        - Thalidomide
    - Environmental Agents
        - Lead
        - Mercury
        - Organic solvents
        - Polychlorinated biphenyls (PCB's)
        - Ionizing radiation
    - Infectious Agents
        - Toxoplasmosis
        - Rubella
        - Cytomegalovirus
        - Syphilis
        - Varicella
- Insulin-dependent diabetes mellitus (IDDM)
- Consanguinity
- Multiple pregnancy losses, stillbirth
- Infertility

Chapter 9 Questions
Fetal Assessment

1. Which of the following is TRUE regarding antenatal screening for anomalies?
   a. In order to ensure cost-effective care, maternal serum alpha-fetoprotein (MSAFP) or triple screening should be offered only to women who have a known risk such as elevated maternal age.
   b. Age, personal and family history, and screening tests should be used as the criteria to identify candidates for complete genetic evaluation.
   c. The triple screen test should be provided between 12 and 15 weeks of pregnancy.
   d. Seventy to eighty percent of all trisomies occur in women over the age of 35, so screening younger women offers limited improvement in the detection of fetal anomalies.

■ **DATA FOR ITEMS 2–4**

As you review the triple screen results of JP, a 38-year-old, obese, G6P4 African-American woman at 18 weeks gestational age, you note that the test was positive for a serum level of alpha-fetoprotein (AFP) elevated above the cutoff value of 2.5 multiples of the mean (MOM).

2. All of the following characteristics of this client can affect the normative levels of alpha-fetoprotein EXCEPT which of the following?
   a. Age
   b. Weight
   c. Race
   d. Parity

3. The results of JP's triple screen alert you to an increased risk of which of the following?
   a. Spina bifida
   b. Down Syndrome
   c. Ectopic pregnancy
   d. Diaphragmatic hernia

4. Which of the following is the BEST next step in the management of this client?
   a. Repeat the triple screen
   b. Confirm the accuracy of the estimated gestational age
   c. Recommend an ultrasound examination
   d. Recommend amniocentesis

5. Which of the following results on a triple screen would alert you to an increased possibility of Down syndrome?
   a. High maternal serum alpha-fetoprotein, high estriol levels, low hCG levels
   b. High maternal serum alpha-fetoprotein, high estriol levels, high hCG levels
   c. Low maternal serum alpha-fetoprotein, low estriol levels, low hCG levels
   d. Low maternal serum alpha-fetoprotein, low estriol levels, high hCG levels

6. To reduce the risk of limb reduction defects related to chorionic villus sampling (CVS) the midwife should recommend which of the following?
   a. The procedure should be performed at approximately 8 weeks gestation.
   b. The procedure should be performed at or after 10 weeks gestation.
   c. The procedure should be performed transcervically.
   d. The procedure should be performed transabdominally.

7. Standard/traditional, genetic amniocentesis is performed at what gestational age?
  a. 8 to 10 weeks gestation
  b. 12 to 14 weeks gestation
  c. 15 to 20 weeks gestation
  d. 20 to 22 weeks gestation

8. Which of the following is NOT a risk of amniocentesis?
  a. Genetic anomalies
  b. Fetal loss
  c. Amnionitis
  d. Isoimunnization

9. What is the MOST common use of amniocentesis in the third trimester?
  a. Rapid karyotyping
  b. Genetic diagnosis
  c. Testing for Rh isoimmunization
  d. Testing for fetal lung maturity

10. Which of the following is NOT a test for fetal lung maturity?
  a. Lecithin/sphingomyelin ratios (L/S)
  b. Phosphatidylglycerol (PG) tests
  c. Optical density assessment of bilirubin in amniotic fluid
  d. The "shake" and "tap" tests

11. Which of the following is TRUE regarding the use of cordocentesis?
  a. It is commonly used instead of amniocentesis for karyotyping.
  b. It is safer than using CVS in third trimester to obtain fetal blood.
  c. It is within the scope of midwifery practice following appropriate training.
  d. It can be used to do fetal blood transfusions or to medicate the fetus.

12. When should fetal movement counting start for women at low risk for uteroplacental insufficiency?
  a. 24 to 26 weeks EGA
  b. 26 to 28 weeks EGA
  c. 30 to 32 weeks EGA
  d. 34 to 36 weeks EGA

13. Which of the following does NOT diminish maternal perception of fetal movement?
  a. Obesity
  b. Polyhydramnios
  c. Oligohydramnios
  d. Anterior placenta

■ **DATA FOR ITEMS 14–15**

YR is a 36-year-old G2P1001 at 36 weeks gestation with an uncomplicated prenatal course. She has come to your office today for an NST due to decreased fetal activity. The NST is reactive.

14. In addition to reinforcing fetal movement counts and sending her home, which of the following is the MOST appropriate management plan for YR?
  a. Tell her that there is no need for serial NST's at this point.
  b. Have her come back in two weeks for another NST.
  c. Have her come back in one week for another NST.
  d. Have her come back in three days for another NST.

■   **ADDITIONAL DATA FOR ITEM 15**

YR calls you back the next day and says that she is really worried because the baby has not moved much since she saw you for the NST the day before. At the conclusion of your phone call, you decide to bring her back for another NST. This time the NST is nonreactive.

15. In addition to consulting with a physician, which of the following is your BEST management plan for YR?

    a. Have her come back next day for evaluation of BPP/AFV

    b. Admit her to the hospital for a probable C-section

    c. Schedule her for immediate BPP/AFV

    d. Repeat the NST to assess the need for additional action

16. Which of the following is TRUE regarding a complete cessation of fetal movements?

    a. It is correlated with impending fetal death.

    b. It is correlated with impending labor.

    c. It is correlated with maternal smoking.

    d. It is correlated with diurnal variations and fetal sleep/wake cycles.

17. Auscultated acceleration tests (ATT) have been proposed as an alternative to which of the following methods of fetal assessment?

    a. Routine auscultation of fetal heart tones throughout pregnancy

    b. Non-stress test

    c. Electronic fetal monitoring during labor

    d. Intermittent auscultation during labor

18. Fetal heart rate reactivity is usually reached at which of the following gestational ages?

    a. 22 to 26 weeks

    b. 26 to 28 weeks

    c. 28 to 32 weeks

    d. 32 to 34 weeks

19. Which of the following statements is TRUE regarding the minimum frequency of serial non-stress tests?

    a. They should be performed at least once every two weeks.

    b. They should be performed at least once every week.

    c. They should be performed bi-weekly (twice a week).

    d. They should be performed every-other day.

20. Which of the following statements is TRUE regarding the frequency of serial nonstress testing for women at particularly high risk for poor outcome related to uteroplacental insufficiency (UPI)?

    a. They should be performed at least once every two weeks.

    b. They should be performed at least once every week.

    c. They should be performed bi-weekly (twice a week).

    d. They should be performed every-other day.

DATA FOR ITEM 21

A 32-year-old G2P1001 at 34 weeks gestation is in to see you for an NST due to gestational diabetes. After 20 minutes, the NST is nonreactive. Her last NST was reactive and she reports normal fetal movement counts over the last couple of days.

21. Which of the following is the BEST step to take next?
   a. Send her home and have her return the next day for a repeat NST when she is well-rested and has just eaten a full meal.
   b. Apply vibroacoustic stimulation (VAS) to stimulate the fetus.
   c. Continue the NST for another 20 to 30 minutes.
   d. Send the woman to the hospital for a BPP or CST.

22. Which of the following methods of fetal assessment is the MOST accurate predictor of uteroplacental insufficiency?
   a. Non-stress test (NST)
   b. Contraction-stress test (CST)
   c. Biophysical profile (BPP)
   d. Amniotic fluid volume (AFV)

23. Which of the following women is NOT a good candidate for a contraction stress test (CST)?
   a. A woman known to have a fetus with intrauterine growth restriction (IUGR)
   b. A woman with a placenta previa
   c. A woman with a previous low-transverse cesarean section
   d. A woman with pregnancy-induced hypertension

24. A contraction-stress test is known to have about a 30 percent false-positive rate. This means which of the following statements is TRUE?
   a. One third of women who have a negative CST have a fetus that is actually normal.
   b. One third of women who have a positive CST have a fetus that is actually normal.
   c. One third of women who have a negative CST have a fetus that is actually compromised.
   d. One third of women who have a positive CST have a fetus that is actually compromised.

DATA FOR ITEM 25

You are performing a contraction stress test (CST) on a 25-year-old G3P1101 who is an insulin-dependent diabetic. You note that she has had six contractions in the last 10 minutes that have lasted an average of 45 seconds. The fetal heart rate demonstrates non-repetitive late decelerations.

25. Which of the following is the MOST appropriate course of action?
   a. Continue the CST until an adequate contraction pattern is established.
   b. Discontinue the CST because there is evidence of hyperstimulation of the uterus.
   c. Consider the test positive (nonreassuring) and arrange for follow-up with a biophysical profile (BPP).
   d. Consider the test equivocal and follow with a BPP or repeat the CST within 24 hours.

26. Which of the following is NOT a criterion of biophysical profile (BPP) scoring?
   a. Placental blood flow
   b. Fetal heart reactivity
   c. Fetal breathing movements
   d. Gross body movement

27. Which of the following are the components of the "modified biophysical profile?"
   a. Fetal breathing movements and nonstress test
   b. Fetal tone and amniotic fluid volume
   c. Fetal tone and fetal breathing movements
   d. Nonstress test and amniotic fluid volume

■   DATA FOR ITEM 28
_____

HD is having a modified biophysical profile. The ultrasonographer has found the following:

Quadrant 1:   1 cm, 2 cm, 4.5 cm pocket of clear amniotic fluid

Quadrant 2:   2.5 cm pocket of clear amniotic fluid

Quadrant 3:   3 cm and 5 cm pocket of clear amniotic fluid

Quadrant 4:   1.5 cm and 5 cm pocket of clear amniotic fluid

28. What is HD's amniotic fluid index (AFI)?
- **a.** 5.0 cm
- **b.** 8.0 cm
- **c.** 17.0 cm
- **d.** 24.5 cm

29. Which of the following is NOT a minimum component of limited obstetrical ultrasound in second and third trimesters?
- **a.** Fetal number
- **b.** Fetal lie
- **c.** Fetal length
- **d.** Fetal cardiac activity

30. The crux of the debate regarding limited versus comprehensive ultrasound examination is best illustrated by which of the following scenarios?
- **a.** A woman wants you to determine the gender of her baby during an ultrasound to screen for fetal anomalies.
- **b.** During an ultrasound in third trimester for size/dates discrepancy, you find out that the baby is anencephalic.
- **c.** During an initial ultrasound to monitor a multiple-gestation pregnancy you determine that there are triplets rather than twins as you had previously thought.
- **d.** During an ultrasound for identification of early fetal heart tones, you miss an ectopic pregnancy.

31. The results of the Routine Antenatal Diagnostic Imaging with Ultrasound (RADIUS) trial to determine whether routine scanning of normal women is appropriate demonstrated which of the following regarding the routine use of ultrasound?
- **a.** Routine ultrasound decreased the rate of maternal and/or neonatal morbidity and mortality.
- **b.** Routine ultrasound increased the rate of induced abortion, amniocentesis, and cesarean section.
- **c.** Routine ultrasound did not affect the rates of maternal and/or neonatal morbidity and mortality.
- **d.** Routine ultrasound decreased the rate of induced abortion, amniocentesis, and cesarean section.

Chapter 9 Answer Key
Fetal Assessment

1. *b* p. 284	**17.** *b* p. 295
2. *d* p. 285	**18.** *c* p. 296
3. *a* p. 285	**19.** *b* p. 297
4. *b* p. 287	**20.** *c* p. 297
5. *d* p. 285–286	**21.** *c* p. 296
6. *b* p. 288	**22.** *b* p. 299
7. *c* p. 289	**23.** *b* p. 299
8. *a* p. 290	**24.** *b* p. 300
9. *d* p. 290	**25.** *d* p. 301
10. *c* p. 290	**26.** *a* p. 302–303
11. *d* p. 290	**27.** *d* p. 304
12. *d* p. 291	**28.** *c* p. 304
13. *a* p. 291	**29.** *c* p. 309
14. *a* p. 291	**30.** *d* p. 308–309
15. *c* p. 294	**31.** *c* p. 311
16. *a* p. 291	

Chapter 10 Outline
Antepartal Complications

I.   Abortion

   A. Induced Abortion

      1. Definition

      2. Management

   B. Spontaneous Abortion

      1. Threatened

         a. Definition

         b. Signs/Symptoms

         c. Management

      2. Inevitable

         a. Definition

         b. Signs/Symptoms

         c. Management

      3. Incomplete

         a. Definition

         b. Signs/Symptoms

         c. Management

      4. Missed

         a. Definition

         b. Signs/Symptoms

         c. Management

   C. Habitual Abortion

      1. Definition

      2. Signs/Symptoms

      3. Management

II.   Incompetent Cervix

   A. Definition

   B. Management

III.   Hydatidiform Mole/Molar Pregnancy

   A. Definition

   B. Signs/Symptoms

   C. Diagnosis

   D. Management

IV.   Ectopic Pregnancy

    A. Definition

    B. Etiology

    C. Predisposing factors

    D. Signs/Symptoms

    E. Diagnosis

    F. Management

V.   Hyperemesis Gravidarium

    A. Definition

    B. Etiology

    C. Predisposing factors

    D. Signs/Symptoms

    E. Management

VI.   Infections in Pregnancy

    A. Urinary Tract Infections (UTI's) in Pregnancy
    Asymptomatic bacteriuria vs. Cystitis vs. Pyelonephritis

        a. Causative agents/Mode of infection

        b. Predisposing factors

        c. Signs/Symptoms

        d. Screening tests/Diagnostic tests

        e. Effects of infection on fetus/neonate

        f. Management/Treatment

    B. Sexually Transmitted Infections/Bacterial Vaginosis/Candidiasis

    (Discussed further in Chapter 2)

        1. Human Immunodeficiency Virus (HIV)

            a. Causative agent/Mode of infection

            b. Predisposing factors

            c. Signs/Symptoms

            d. Screening tests/Diagnostic tests

                i. ELISA/Western Blot

                ii. Viral Cultures

                iii. Polymerase Chain Reaction (RPR)

                iv. P24 Antigen Assays

                v. CD4 Counts

                vi. Effects of infection on fetus/neonate

                vii. Management/Treatment

                    a. CDC Guidelines for Antiretroviral Therapy in Pregnancy and Labor

                    b. CDC Guidelines for Antiretroviral Therapy in Neonates

C. Group B Streptococcus (GBS)
   1. Causative agent/Mode of infection
   2. Signs/Symptoms
   3. Screening tests/Diagnostic tests
   4. Effects of infection on fetus/neonate
   5. Management/Treatment
      a. CDC Prevention Strategies for early-onset GBS (prenatal screening vs. risk factor approaches)

D. Tuberculosis
   1. Causative agent/Mode of infection
   2. Signs/Symptoms
   3. Screening tests/Diagnostic tests
      a. Mantoux test/Purified protein derivative (PPD)
      b. Anergy panel
   4. Effects of infection on fetus/neonate
   5. Management/Treatment

E. Hepatitis A, B, C
   1. Causative agents/Mode of infection
   2. Predisposing factors
   3. Signs/Symptoms
   4. Screening tests/Diagnostic tests
      Antigen tests vs. antibody tests
   5. Effects of infection on fetus/neonate
   6. Management/Treatment/Vaccination

F. Cytomegalovirus (CMV)
   1. Causative agent/Mode of infection
   2. Signs/Symptoms
   3. Screening tests/Diagnostic tests
   4. Effects of infection on fetus/neonate
   5. Management

G. Toxoplasmosis
   1. Causative agent/Mode of infection
   2. Signs/Symptoms
   3. Screening tests/Diagnostic tests
   4. Effects of infection on fetus/neonate
   5. Management/Treatment

H. Varicella
   1. Causative agent/Mode of infection
   2. Signs/Symptoms
   3. Screening tests/Diagnostic tests
   4. Effects of infection on fetus/neonate
   5. Management/Treatment/Vaccinations

I. Rubella
  1. Causative agent/Mode of infection
  2. Signs/Symptoms
  3. Screening tests/Diagnostic tests
  4. Effects of infection on fetus/neonate
  5. Management/Treatment/Vaccination

J. Listeria
  1. Causative agent/Mode of infection
  2. Signs/Symptoms
  3. Screening tests/Diagnostic tests
  4. Effects of infection on fetus/neonate
  5. Management/Treatment

K. Measles (Rubeola)
  1. Causative agent/Mode of infection
  2. Signs/Symptoms
  3. Screening tests/Diagnostic tests
  4. Effects of infection on fetus/neonate
  5. Management/Treatment/Vaccination

L. Parvovirus (Fifth Disease)
  1. Causative agent/Mode of infection
  2. Signs/Symptoms
  3. Screening tests/Diagnostic tests
  4. Effects of infection on fetus/neonate
  5. Management/Treatment

VII. **Hematologic Disorders**

  A. ABO Incompatibility/Irregular Antibodies
    1. Definition
    2. Etiology
    3. Screening tests/Diagnostic tests
    4. Effects on fetus/neonate
        Hemolytic disease of the newborn

  B. Rh (D) Incompatibility/Isoimmunization
    1. Definition
    2. Etiology
    3. Screening tests/Diagnostic tests
      a. Indirect vs Direct Coomb's Tests
    4. Effects on fetus/neonate
      a. Hemolytic disease of the newborn
      b. Erythroblastosis fetalis/Hydrops fetalis

      5. Management/Treatment

        a. D immunoglobulin (RhoGam)

   C. Thalassemia (Alpha vs. Beta Thalessemia)

      1. Definition

      2. Etiology

      3. Signs/Symptoms

      4. Screening tests/Diagnostic tests

        Hemoglobin electrophoresis

      5. Effects on fetus/neonate

      6. Management

   D. Anemia

      1. Definition

      2. Etiology

        Iron vs. Folate vs. Vitamin B_{12} deficiencies

          Microcytic/Normocytic/Macrocytic Anemias

      3. Predisposing factors

      4. Signs/Symptoms

      5. Screening tests/Diagnostic tests and criteria

      6. Effects on fetus/neonate

      7. Obstetrical complications associated with anemia

      8. Management/Treatment

   E. Glucose–6-Phosphate Dehydrogenase (G6PD) Deficiency

      1. Definition

      2. Etiology

      3. Signs/Symptoms

      4. Screening tests/Diagnostic tests

      5. Effects on fetus/neonate

      6. Management

   F. Hemoglobin S/Sickle Cell Trait/Sickle Cell Disease

      1. Definition

      2. Etiology

      3. Signs/Symptoms

      4. Screening tests/Diagnostic tests

        a. Sickledex/Sickle prep

        b. Hemoglobin electrophoresis

      5. Effects on fetus/neonate

      6. Management

VIII. Asthma

   A. Definition

   B. Etiology

   C. Predisposing factors

   D. Signs /Symptoms

E. Screening tests/Diagnostic tests

F. Management/Treatment

IX. **Gestational Diabetes Mellitus (GDM)**

  A. Definition

  B. Etiology

  C. Predisposing factors

  D. Signs/Symptoms

  E. Screening tests/Diagnostic tests
    1. Glucose finger stick
    2. 1-hour glucose challenge test
    3. 3-hour glucose tolerance test (GTT)

  F. Effects on fetus/neonate

  G. Obstetrical complications associated with GDM

  H. Management/Treatment
    1. Nutrition
    2. Exercise
    3. Insulin

X. **Thyroid Disorders (Hyperthyroid vs. Hypothyroid)**

  A. Definition

  B. Etiology

  C. Signs/Symptoms

  D. Screening tests/Diagnostic tests

  E. Effects on fetus/neonate

  F. Management

XI. **Multiple Gestation Pregnancy**

  A. Signs/Symptoms

  B. Obstetrical complications associated with multiple gestation pregnancy

  C. Management

XII. **Polyhydramnios**

  A. Definition

  B. Etiology

  C. Signs/Symptoms

  D. Diagnostic tests

  E. Obstetrical complications associated with polyhydramnios

  F. Management

XIII. Oligohydramnios

A. Definition

B. Etiology

C. Signs/Symptoms

D. Diagnostic tests

E. Obstetrical complications associated with oligohydramnios

F. Management

XIV. Fetal Death

A. Etiology

B. Signs/Symptoms

C. Obstetric complications associated with fetal death
1. Disseminated intravascular coagulation
2. Amniotic fluid embolism

D. Management

XV. Hypertensive Disorders of Pregnancy

(Preeclampsia/Eclampsia/Chronic Hypertension/Chronic Hypertension with Superimposed Preeclampsia/Transient Hypertension)

A. Definition

B. Etiology

C. Predisposing factors

D. Signs/Symptoms

E. Screening tests/Diagnostic tests

F. Obstetrical complications associated with hypertension

G. Management/Treatment
Magnesium Sulfate therapy

XVI. Antepartal Bleeding (Placenta Previa/Abruptio Placenta)

(See Table 1 at the end of this section for "Differential Diagnosis for Antepartal Bleeding")

A. Definition

B. Etiology

C. Predisposing factors

D. Signs/Symptoms

E. Diagnostic tests/exams
Double set-up exam

F. Obstetrical complications associated with placenta previa/abruptio placenta

G. Management

XVII. Size-Dates Discrepancy

A. Definition

B. Etiology

C. Signs/Symptoms
1. Fundal height measurement
2. Leopold's maneuvers

D. Diagnosis

E. Management

XVIII. Intrauterine Growth Retardation (IUGR)/Small-for-Gestational-Age (SGA)

A. Definition

B. Etiology

C. Predisposing factors

D. Signs/Symptoms

E. Diagnosis

F. Management

XIX. Large-for-Gestational-Age (LGA)/Macrosomia

A. Definition

B. Etiology

C. Signs/symptoms

D. Diagnosis

E. Obstetrical complications associated with LGA

F. Management

XX. Postdates Pregnancy

A. Definition

B. Etiology

C. Obstetrical complications associated with postdates pregnancy
Postmaturity syndrome

D. Management
1. Fetal movement counts
2. Non-stress tests (NST)
3. Contraction stress test (CST)
4. Amniotic fluid volume/Amniotic fluid index (AFI)

■   **Table 1**   **Differential Diagnosis for Antepartal Bleeding**

- Vaginitis
- Cervicitis
- Spontaneous abortion
- Implantation bleeding
- Ruptured uterus
- Bloody show
- Placenta previa
- Abruptio placenta
- Hydatidiform mole
- Ectopic pregnancy
- Cervical erosion
- Cervical cancer
- Cervical polyps
- Recent cone biopsy
- Ruptured vaginal septum
- Ruptured vaginal or vulvar varicosities
- Vaginal trauma
- Condylomata acuminata
- Rectal hemorrhoids
- Rectal polyps
- Rectal cancer
- Urethritis
- Hemorrhagic cystitis
- Extrachorial placentas
- Ruptured vasa previa

Chapter 10 Questions
Antepartal Complications

1. Which of the following scenarios presents the WORST prognosis for continuation of pregnancy in the first trimester?
   a. Postcoital vaginal bleeding
   b. Vaginal bleeding and uterine size less than dates
   c. Vaginal bleeding and cramping abdominal pain
   d. Vaginal bleeding at a date after fetal heart activity is first detected

■ **DATA FOR ITEMS 2–3**

TG is a 26-year-old G3P1021 at approximately 9 weeks gestational age by LMP. She calls you at 3:30 a.m. because when she went to the bathroom she noticed some blood on her underwear. She describes the bleeding as a "couple of spots the size of dimes." She denies any abdominal or back pain and has no symptoms of a urinary tract infection. You have her take her temperature and call you back. When she returns your call she states that her temperature is 99.1°F. She also states that she is concerned because she has had more light bleeding since you spoke and begins to cry and say "this is just like the last time I had a miscarriage."

2. Which of the following is your BEST course of action at this time?
   a. Have her come in to the hospital for a pelvic exam, possible ultrasound, and further evaluation.
   b. Have her come in to the hospital and inform your consulting physician so that she is familiar with the patient and the clinical situation.
   c. Recommend pelvic rest, teach her the symptoms that need to be reported immediately, and have her keep her appointment one week from today.
   d. Recommend pelvic rest, teach her the symptoms that need to be reported immediately, and have her come in to the office the next day.

■ **ADDITIONAL DATA FOR ITEM 3**

When you next see TG, you perform a gentle speculum exam and find no signs of vaginitis or cervicitis. You do note some pooling of fresh (bright red) blood in the posterior fornix. Her vital signs are within normal limits and her bimanual exam is also within normal limits. She does not have any cramping or pain. She is extremely emotionally distressed.

3. Which of the following actions is MOST appropriate at this time?
   a. Obtain an ultrasound evaluation within 24 hours.
   b. Order serial quantitative serum hCG levels.
   c. Send her home after reiterating the need for pelvic rest and reviewing symptoms that should be reported.
   d. Inform your consulting physician of your findings so that she is familiar with the patient and the clinical situation.

4. For how long should sexual intercourse be avoided following a first trimester spontaneous abortion?
   a. 1 to 2 weeks
   b. 2 to 4 weeks
   c. 4 to 6 weeks
   d. 6 to 8 weeks

5. A client who has just experienced a first trimester spontaneous abortion asks you why she needs to wait to resume sexual intercourse. Which of the following is the MOST accurate response?

   a. Because the tissue is traumatized and bleeding could resume
   b. Because pregnancy is possible and the uterus needs time to heal before another pregnancy occurs
   c. Because there is an increased risk of infection at this time
   d. Because the uterus is irritable and painful cramping can occur following orgasm

6. A woman is said to suffer from habitual abortions when spontaneous abortion has terminated the course of how many pregnancies?

   a. Two or more consecutive
   b. Three or more at any time
   c. Three or more consecutive
   d. Four or more at any time

7. Which of the following statements is TRUE regarding the timing of a pregnancy loss due to incompetent cervix?

   a. It is most likely to occur late in the first trimester.
   b. It is most likely to occur in the second trimester.
   c. It is most likely to occur early in the third trimester.
   d. It is equally likely at any stage in pregnancy.

8. Which of the following is NOT a risk factor for incompetent cervix?

   a. Previous cervical cone biopsy
   b. History of a cervical laceration during previous childbirth
   c. Previous fetal losses due to uterine congenital anomalies
   d. History of three or more abortions using suction

DATA FOR ITEM 9

You are performing a vaginal speculum and digital examination on a woman who has had a Modified Shirodkar cerclage procedure. Her estimated gestational age is 22 weeks.

9. Which of the following findings on examination is an indication for removal of the sutures?

   a. Breech presentation
   b. Sixty percent effacement of the cervix
   c. Vaginal bleeding
   d. Rupture of membranes without labor

10. Which of the following is NOT a usual site for an ectopic pregnancy?

   a. Cervix
   b. Ovaries
   c. Fallopian tube
   d. Vaginal wall

DATA FOR ITEM 11

A 22 year-old G2P1011 comes to see you because she has had vaginal spotting for 5 days and now presents with significant pain in her lower right abdominal area. Her last menstrual period was approximately 6 weeks ago. She does not have a fever.

11. Which of the following should you do FIRST in assessing this client?

   a. Pelvic exam for uterine sizing/adenexal masses and early ultrasound
   b. Pelvic exam for uterine sizing/adenexal masses and qualitative hCG
   c. Ultrasound and single quantitative serum hCG
   d. Ultrasound and repeated qualitative serum hCG

12. Following the diagnosis of an ectopic pregnancy, which of the following is the MOST appropriate management step?

    a. Obtain a transvaginal ultrasound to confirm diagnosis

    b. Counsel the woman on her options: surgery or medical management with methotrexate

    c. Admit to the hospital

    d. Refer immediately to physician for management

13. Which of the following is NOT a predisposing risk factor for an ectopic pregnancy?

    a. Intrauterine contraceptive devices

    b. Bilateral tubal ligation

    c. Pelvic infections

    d. Two or more induced abortions

DATA FOR ITEMS 14–15

VS is a 40-year-old G4P2103 at 15 weeks estimated gestational age (EGA) by LMP. This is VS's first prenatal visit. She presents with some bloody vaginal discharge that has been intermittent for the last week. She also complains of daily nausea and vomiting. She has had no abdominal pain or cramping. On your abdominal exam you find a large-for-dates uterus, but you cannot find a fetal heart tone. The speculum exam is unremarkable for the exception of some brownish bloody discharge. On bimanual exam you find that she has some adnexal tenderness. Her cervix is long, closed and posterior.

14. Which of the following is the MOST likely diagnosis?

    a. Threatened abortion

    b. Ectopic pregnancy

    c. Hydatidiform mole

    d. Multiple gestation

15. Which of the following would be MOST helpful in confirming your diagnosis?

    a. Sonogram

    b. Serial serum quantitative hCG levels

    c. Single serum quantitative hCG level and sonogram

    d. Serial serum quantitative hCG levels and sonogram

16. Which of the following is diagnostic for tuberculosis?

    a. Rales on auscultation

    b. Pleurisy with effusion

    c. Positive Mantoux test (purified protein derivative test or PPD)

    d. Positive chest x-ray

DATA FOR ITEM 17

CE has come to see you for her initial prenatal visit. She is originally from Jamaica and states that she received a bacillus Calmette-Guerin (BCG) vaccination as a child. You note in her chart that she had a negative chest x-ray 4 years ago.

17. Which of the following would be the MOST appropriate management of this client?

    a. Administer a Mantoux test (PPD) to establish whether she is immune

    b. Readminister the BCG vaccine to ensure continued immunity

    c. Repeat the chest x-ray

    d. Obtain serum titers to assess immune status

DATA FOR ITEMS 18–19

VR is a 28-year-old G3P1011 migrant farm-worker from El Salvador at 16 weeks estimated gestational age (EGA). She has come in to have her Mantoux test read four days after you administered the purified protein derivative (PPD). You note that there is some reddening in the area as well as an area of palpable swelling that measures approximately 12 mm. Her Mantoux test with her previous pregnancy 2 years earlier was negative. She has no signs or symptoms of active tuberculosis.

18. Which of the following is the MOST accurate interpretation of this test result?
    a. It cannot be evaluated because it is more than 72 hours since the PPD was administered.
    b. It can be evaluated and it is considered positive because she has risk factors for tuberculosis.
    c. It can be evaluated and it is considered negative because the induration is not at least 15 mm in diameter.
    d. It cannot be evaluated because there is a high chance that she has been vaccinated previously with bacillus Calmette-Guerin (BCG).

19. What is the BEST step to take next in the management of this patient?
    a. Order a sputum culture
    b. Order a chest x-ray
    c. Order a sputum culture and chest x-ray
    d. Order a repeat Mantoux test to be evaluated within 72 hours

20. Which of the following statements is TRUE regarding the use of isoniazid (INH) treatment in pregnancy?
    a. INH use in pregnancy has been approved by the FDA.
    b. INH treatment is recommended for prophylaxis in all pregnant women with a positive Mantoux test and a negative chest x-ray.
    c. Most clinicians recommend continuation of INH treatment or prophylaxis if a woman becomes pregnant during a treatment course to avoid drug resistance.
    d. INH has been shown to be teratogenic so treatment and prophylaxis for tuberculosis should be postponed until after delivery.

21. Which of the following types of viral hepatitis is transmitted via the fecal-oral route?
    a. Hepatitis A
    b. Hepatitis B
    c. Hepatitis C
    d. Hepatitis D

22. Which of the following statements regarding maternal-infant transmission of Hepatitis B is TRUE?
    a. Vertical transmission of Hepatitis B to the fetus is very rare, but has serious implications.
    b. Transmission of Hepatitis B to the fetus is more common during Cesarean section than during vaginal birth.
    c. Hepatitis B can be transmitted enterally or parenterally.
    d. Hepatitis B virus is present in all of an infected woman's body fluids except breast milk.

23. Which of the following statements regarding Hepatitis A is TRUE?
    a. It has a slow, invidious onset and prolonged acute phase.
    b. It commonly results in both a chronic and carrier states of the disease.
    c. No adverse fetal effects of active maternal infection have been identified.
    d. Vertical transmission is common but pregnancy outcome is not affected.

24. Which of the following is TRUE regarding a positive result on Hepatitis B Surface Antigen (HBsAg) screening test?
    a. It could be positive due to previous immunization with either Hepatitis B vaccine or Hepatitis B immune globulin (HBIG).
    b. It indicates active Hepatitis B infection (acute or chronic) only.
    c. It could represent either current/active or prior/non-active infection with Hepatitis B.
    d. It indicates that the body has, at some point, mounted an immune response to Hepatitis B.

25. Which of the following represents the BEST management of the newborn infants of Hepatitis B-infected mothers?

   a. Immediate bath, immunization with Hepatitis B immune globulin (HBIG), and immunization with Hepatitis B vaccine

   b. Immediate bath, blood draw to determine infection status, immunization with Hepatitis B immune globulin (HBIG), immunization with Hepatitis B vaccine pending blood work results

   c. Immediate bath, postponing of breastfeeding until acute maternal infection resolves, immunization with Hepatitis B vaccine only

   d. Immediate bath, postponing of breastfeeding until acute maternal infection resolves, immunization with both Hepatitis B immune globulin (HBIG) and with Hepatitis B vaccine

■ DATA FOR ITEM 26

RT is a 34-year-old G1P0 who became infected with Hepatitis C following a transfusion to treat injuries sustained after a motor vehicle accident three years ago. She wants to know how the disease will affect the care she receives in pregnancy and birth.

26. Which of the following is the BEST answer to RT's question?

   a. That her care will be transferred to a physician both for pregnancy and birth

   b. That she will be monitored for signs of abnormal liver disease that may affect her nutritional status

   c. That she and her newborn will both receive Hepatitis C immune globulin close to delivery to help prevent transmission

   d. That her newborn will receive Hepatitis C immune globulin and Hepatitis C vaccine

27. In which of the following stages of pregnancy is maternal infection with rubella MOST likely to cause congenital malformations?

   a. Anytime in the first trimester

   b. In the first month

   c. Anytime in the third trimester

   d. In the last month

28. Which of the following is the BEST description of the rash characteristic of rubella infection?

   a. Slow-spreading and composed primarily of vesicles that break open and then crust over

   b. Pale or bright red, spreading rapidly from face to entire body, and then fading rapidly

   c. Pale red on the face giving the appearance of a "slapped cheek"

   d. Umbilicated lesions predominantly on the palms of hands and soles of feet

■ DATA FOR ITEM 29

A woman comes to see you because she received a rubella vaccination two weeks ago and has just found out that she is approximately 4 weeks pregnant.

29. What is the MOST appropriate action at this time?

   a. Inform the woman that the vaccine is a known teratogen and then help her explore her options to either continue or terminate the pregnancy.

   b. Inform the woman that due to the timing of when she received the vaccination, that her fetus has a 50 percent risk of being born with congenital malformations.

   c. Explain to the woman that there is a theoretical risk from the vaccine but that there is no demonstrated evidence of teratogenicity from the vaccine.

   d. Explain to her that there is a 20 percent risk of congenital malformations and that you will have to wait for three months to draw her antibody titer to determine infection status.

30. Which of the following is the MOST accurate set of instructions on ways to avoid toxoplasmosis?
    a. Avoid contact with cat feces, wear gloves while gardening, avoid eating raw or undercooked meat
    b. Avoid contacts with cats, avoid gardening in areas where cats defecate, avoid eating raw or undercooked meat
    c. Avoid contact with cat feces, avoid contact with individuals with active toxoplasmosis, avoid eating raw or undercooked meat
    d. Avoid contact with cat feces, wear gloves while gardening, avoid raw or undercooked fish

31. In which stage of pregnancy is maternal infection with varicella MOST likely to cause congenital varicella syndrome in the fetus?
    a. The first 20 weeks
    b. The second trimester
    c. The last 6 weeks
    d. The last 2 weeks

32. What is the MOST common cause of maternal mortality related to varicella?
    a. Varicella pneumonia
    b. Disseminated varicella infection
    c. Chorioamnionitis
    d. Hydronephrosis

■ DATA FOR ITEMS 33–34

MQ is a 29-year-old G1P0 at approximately 39 $^{+2}$ weeks gestational age. Her prenatal course has been unremarkable except for the fact that she does not have immunity to varicella and was exposed to the virus two weeks ago. You administered one dose of varicella-zoster immune globulin (VZIG) at that time. She calls you today because she has had a fever, chills, and muscle pain for the last two days and is worried. She has an appointment to see you later that day.

33. What is your BEST course of action at this time in the management of this woman's care?
    a. Have her come in to your office as scheduled for a serologic varicella antibody test and possible acyclovir treatment
    b. Have her come in to your office as scheduled for varicella vaccine
    c. Have her come in to your office after office hours for serologic varicella antibody test and physical exam
    d. Have her come in to your office after office hours for physical exam and counseling/education

■ ADDITIONAL DATA FOR ITEM 34

Two days later, MQ develops a vesicular rash on her head and neck with occasional vesicle on her abdomen. Despite efforts to postpone delivery, MQ goes into labor on the fourth day after eruption of the vesicles and delivers a 7 lb 12 oz. male infant with no signs of distress or of varicella infection.

34. What is your BEST course of action at this time in the management of the postpartum care of this woman and infant?
    a. Give VZIG to the mother and the infant and isolate the infant from the mother
    b. Give VZIG to the mother and the infant and isolate the mother and the infant together
    c. Give vaccine to the mother and VZIG to the infant and isolate the infant from the mother
    d. Give VZIG to the infant immediately and consider isolation of infant from mother

35. Which of the following physiological changes of pregnancy makes pregnant women more susceptible to urinary tract infections?
   a. Hydronephrosis, which causes urinary stasis
   b. Change in vaginal bacterial flora and thus changes in vaginal pH
   c. Change in urine pH that makes urine more hospitable to microorganisms
   d. Mechanical friction of expanding uterus and presenting part on the urethra

36. Which of the following results of a urine bacterial counts indicates the presence of a urinary tract infection?
   a. 10,000 bacteria of same species per milliliter of urine
   b. 30,000 mixed bacteria per milliliter of urine
   c. 50,000 bacteria of same species per milliliter of urine
   d. 100,000 mixed bacteria per milliliter of urine

37. A black woman with recurrent urinary tract infections should FIRST be screened for which of the following?
   a. Hydronephritis
   b. Sickle cell trait/disease
   c. Thalassemia major
   d. Pernicious anemia

38. Which of the following is NOT a sequela of untreated asymptomatic bacteriuria in pregnancy?
   a. Low birth weight infant
   b. Diabetes mellitus
   c. Pyelonephritis
   d. Preterm labor

DATA FOR ITEMS 39–40

TF is a 36-year-old G3P1101 at approximately 29 weeks gestational age. During her first pregnancy she had recurrent urinary tract infections and preterm labor and delivery at 30 weeks. Based on her history, you ordered repeat urine cultures each trimester. The laboratory results of her 28 week urinalysis and culture suggest that TF has asymptomatic bacteriuria. You treated her with a 10-day course of ampicillin.

39. When is it MOST appropriate to have TF come back for a follow-up urine culture to test for the effectiveness of the ampicillin treatment?
   a. In one week
   b. In ten days
   c. In two weeks
   d. In three weeks

ADDITIONAL DATA FOR ITEM 40

The test of cure on TF's urine specimen shows that there is continuing infection.

40. Which of the following is the BEST course of action at this time?
   a. Obtain a careful history of compliance with treatment regime and prescribe her another course of ampicillin.
   b. Obtain a careful history of compliance with treatment regime and prescribe another course of treatment with a different drug based on sensitivity testing.
   c. Order another test of cure urine culture in case this one was either contaminated or in case the medicine had not had long enough to eradicate the infection.
   d. Commence suppressive therapy and continue it throughout the rest of pregnancy.

41. When would it be MOST appropriate to initiate suppressive therapy for asymptomatic bacteriuria?
    a. When one complete course of treatment has been completed without a cure
    b. When two complete courses of treatment have been completed without a cure
    c. When three complete courses of treatment have been completed without a cure
    d. When four complete courses of treatment have been completed without a cure

42. Which of the following women should NOT receive a nitrofurantoin drug to treat asymptomatic bacteriuria?
    a. A woman near term
    b. A woman with sickle cell disease
    c. A woman with anemia
    d. A woman with a glucose-6-phosphate dehydrogenase (G6PD) deficiency

43. Which of the following is NOT an expected finding from microscopic urinalysis of a woman with cystitis?
    a. Bacteriuria
    b. Hematuria
    c. Dysuria
    d. Pyuria

44. Which of the following is the most common cause of true anemia during pregnancy?
    a. Physiological changes in plasma and red cell production
    b. Iron deficiency
    c. Folate deficiency
    d. Increased iron demands

45. Which of the following BEST describes hemodilution of pregnancy?
    a. Normal increase in plasma volume that outpaces increase in erythrocyte production
    b. Pathological increase in plasma volume that outpaces increase in erythrocyte production
    c. Normal increase in plasma volume with a decrease in the rate of erythrocyte production
    d. Pathological increase in plasma volume with a decrease in the rate of erythrocyte production

46. Which of the following is the generally accepted, working definition of anemia in pregnant women?
    a. Hemoglobin level less than 14.0 g per 100 mL (14 g/dL)
    b. Hemoglobin level less than 12.0 g per 100 mL (12 g/dL)
    c. Hemoglobin level less than 10.0 g per 100 mL (10 g/dL)
    d. Hemoglobin level less than 9.0 g per 100 mL (9 g/dL)

■   **DATA FOR ITEMS 47–48**

The laboratory results of GH, a 16-year-old G1P0 at her initial prenatal visit at an estimated 8 weeks gestational age, reveal that her hemoglobin is 10 g/dL. You note that her medical chart states that she suffered from bulimia at the age of 14. GH is currently asymptomatic for anemia and denies any bingeing and purging. She is of normal weight for her height.

47. What is the BEST management option for GH at this point?
    a. Nutritional counseling and a referral for a psychiatric consult
    b. Iron, folic acid, and vitamin supplementation and nutritional counseling
    c. Iron, folic acid, and vitamin supplementation and a repeat CBC with differential
    d. Nutritional counseling and consult with MD for further evaluation

PART III

■ ADDITIONAL DATA FOR ITEM 48

You see GH again 8 weeks later and her hemoglobin at this time is 11 g/DL. She has no complaints at this time other than the fact that the iron supplements have caused her to become constipated.

48. What is your BEST course of action at this time?

    a. Continue iron supplementation, provide advice on relief measures for constipation, and re-evaluate hemoglobin level at 28 weeks gestation

    b. Change the iron formulation to one that has fewer GI side effects, continue supplementation, and re-evaluate hemoglobin level in one week

    c. Increase iron supplementation because response to therapy has not been adequate, provide advice on relief measures for constipation, and re-evaluate hemoglobin in two weeks

    d. Continue iron supplementation, provide advice on relief measures for constipation , and order more specific blood indices (such as ferritin and transferrin levels) to assess cause for inadequate response

49. What is the daily recommended amount of elemental iron supplementation in pregnancy?

    a. 30 mg

    b. 60 mg

    c. 90 mg

    d. 120 mg

■ DATA FOR ITEM 50

The following are the results of an initial laboratory evaluation for anemia of LD, a 22-year-old G3P1011 at 20 weeks gestation: Hemoglobin 9.8 g/dL; low reticulocyte count; and a mean corpuscular volume (MCV) of 98.

50. These results suggest which of the following?

    a. Macrocytic anemia

    b. Microcytic anemia

    c. Hemolytic anemia

    d. Aplastic anemia

■ DATA FOR ITEM 51

HG is a 23-year-old G2P0; the result of her hemoglobin electrophoresis reveals that she has hemoglobin (Hb) AS.

51. Which of the following statements is TRUE regarding HG's hemoglobin electrophoresis result?

    a. It shows that she has sickle cell disease.

    b. It shows that she has sickle cell trait.

    c. It shows that she has beta thalassemia.

    d. It shows that she has normal hemoglobin.

52. Which of the following is TRUE regarding the prenatal care of a woman with sickle cell trait?

    a. Because anemia is more likely, you should order a CBC with differential every trimester.

    b. Because of the possibility of a sickle cell crisis, you should manage this woman's care in collaboration with a physician.

    c. You do not need to make any adaptations for the prenatal care of women with sickle cell trait.

    d. Because urinary tract infections are more likely, you should monitor her closely for asymptomatic bacteriuria.

DATA FOR ITEMS 53–54

RD is a 21-year-old at approximately 8 weeks gestational age with sickle cell trait. You have just informed her that the hemoglobin electrophoresis lab results for the father of her baby revealed that he is also a sickle cell trait carrier. The woman asks you what the chances are that her baby will have sickle cell disease.

53. What is the MOST accurate answer to RD's question?
   a. Her infant has a one in ten (1/10) chance of having sickle cell disease.
   b. Her infant has a one in four (1/4) chance of having sickle cell disease.
   c. Her infant has a one in two (1/2) chance of having sickle cell disease.
   d. You cannot give her an accurate probability because there are various factors involved in the development of the disease.

54. What is the BEST management plan for RD?
   a. Transfer her care to a physician knowledgeable in the management of complex hematologic problems
   b. Discuss the risks and benefits of prenatal diagnosis and of various treatment options
   c. Repeat the hemoglobin electrophoresis due to a high rate of false positives
   d. Schedule an appointment for RD with a genetic counselor

---

DATA FOR ITEM 55

PQ, a woman with sickle cell disease, is thinking about getting pregnant. She comes to see you for preconceptual counseling and asks you whether pregnancy will affect the course of the disease.

55. Which is the BEST response to PQ's question?
   a. That pregnancy increases the frequency but not the intensity of sickle cell crises
   b. That pregnancy increased the intensity but not the frequency of sickle cell crises
   c. That pregnancy increases both the intensity and the frequency of sickle cell crises
   d. That pregnancy does not change the frequency or intensity of sickle cell crises

56. Which of the following women would be MOST likely to have glucose–6-phosphate dehyrogenase (G6PD) deficiency?
   a. A woman of Japanese descent
   b. A woman of Guatemalan descent
   c. A woman of Turkish descent
   d. A woman of German descent

57. During pregnancy, when does cardiac output peak, making it most likely for a woman with cardiac disease to decompensate?
   a. At 16 to 20 weeks
   b. At 20 to 24 weeks
   c. At 24 to 28 weeks
   d. At 28 to 32 weeks

58. What is the BEST response to a woman who asks whether being pregnant will affect her asthma?
   a. Pregnancy makes asthma worse
   b. Pregnancy makes asthma better
   c. Pregnancy neither improves nor worsens asthma
   d. The clinical course of asthma in pregnancy cannot be predicted

59. Asthma is NOT associated with which of the following complications?
   a. Trophoblastic disease
   b. Hyperemesis gravidarium
   c. Preeclampsia
   d. Low birth weight

60. Which of the following medications should be avoided in the pregnant asthmatic patient?
   a. Pitocin
   b. Terbutaline
   c. Hemabate
   d. Metoclopramide

61. When in pregnancy should a woman with no identified risk factors for diabetes mellitus be screened for gestational diabetes?
   a. At the initial visit only
   b. At 28 weeks gestation
   c. During first trimester and at 28 weeks gestation
   d. At 28 weeks gestation and at 36 weeks gestation

62. Which of the following is NOT a primary risk factor for gestational diabetes?
   a. Family history of diabetes mellitus
   b. Large-for-gestational-age fetus in this pregnancy
   c. Recurrent glycosuria
   d. Gestational diabetes in a previous pregnancy

63. Why should a fasting blood sugar NOT be used as the sole screening criteria in pregnancy?
   a. Because the fasting blood sugar in gestational diabetics may be normal
   b. Because the fasting blood sugar in gestational diabetics is low
   c. Because the fasting blood sugar in gestational diabetics is high
   d. Because there is a normal physiological elevation of fasting blood sugar in pregnancy

DATA FOR ITEM 64

The serum blood sugar level of a prenatal client following a non-fasting, 1-hour, 50g glucose screening test at 28 weeks gestation was 140 mg per 100 mL of plasma.

64. Which of the following is the MOST appropriate action at this time?
   a. Nothing, this level is within normal
   b. Rescreen at 34–36 weeks gestation
   c. Diagnose this client as a diabetic and consult with a physician
   d. Order a 3-hour glucose tolerance test (GTT)

65. Which of the following complications is NOT caused by gestational diabetes mellitus?
   a. Macrosomia
   b. Shoulder dystocia
   c. Operative delivery
   d. Congenital malformations

DATA FOR ITEM 66

The following are the results of a 3-hour glucose tolerance test (GTT) of a woman at 30 weeks gestation with no risk factors for GDM other than a positive 1-hour glucose challenge screening test:

Fasting	100 mg of glucose per 100 mL of plasma
1 hour	200 mg of glucose per 100 mL of plasma
2 hour	150 mg of glucose per 100 mL of plasma
3 hour	130 mg of glucose per 100 mL of plasma

66. Which of the following is the BEST interpretation and management of these results?
   a. This client is a gestational diabetic; initiate nutritional interventions and blood glucose monitoring.
   b. This client is not a gestational diabetic; continue routine prenatal care.
   c. This client has borderline test results; a repeat test should be done as soon as possible.
   d. This client has borderline test results; you should rescreen this client at 34 weeks.

67. Which of the following is NOT an appropriate intervention to manage gestational diabetes?
    a. Exercise in those without a medical or obstetrical contraindication
    b. Home blood glucose monitoring
    c. Insulin
    d. Oral hypoglycemic agents

68. A woman with gestational diabetes is at an increased risk for which of the following?
    a. Development of Type II diabetes
    b. Oligohydramnios
    c. Uterine rupture
    d. Post dates pregnancy

69. Which of the following is the tocolytic of choice to treat preterm labor in multiple pregnancy?
    a. Magnesium sulfate
    b. Terbutaline
    c. Indomethacin
    d. Nifedipine

70. Which of the following statements is TRUE regarding indirect Coomb's testing?
    a. It tests fetal blood for Rh type
    b. It tests maternal blood for Rh type
    c. It tests fetal blood for Rh antibodies
    d. It tests maternal blood for Rh antibodies

71. A woman who is Rh negative has a negative indirect Coomb's test at 28 weeks. What is the MOST appropriate management at this time?
    a. Order a direct Coomb's test
    b. Administer 300 mcg of Rh immune globulin (RhoGAM)
    c. Consult with a physician for management
    d. Order a Kleinhauer-Betke test to identify fetal blood cells in maternal circulation

72. For how long does Rh immune globulin (RhoGAM) provide protection against developing Rh antibodies?
    a. 10 weeks
    b. 12 weeks
    c. 14 weeks
    d. 16 weeks

73. Which of the following is NOT associated with the development of oligohydramnios?
    a. Congenital anomalies
    b. Intrauterine growth retardation
    c. Erythroblastosis fetalis
    d. Postmature syndrome

74. Which of the following BEST describes the normal changes in amniotic fluid volume during pregnancy?
    a. A gradual increase throughout pregnancy with a peak at term
    b. A gradual increase through 33 to 35 weeks gestation and then a decrease until term
    c. A gradual increase through 33 to 35 weeks gestation and then a plateau until term
    d. A gradual increase until term and then a decrease in a postdates pregnancy

75. Which of the following complications is NOT associated with polyhydramnios?
   a. Cord prolapse
   b. Postmaturity syndrome
   c. Placental abruption
   d. Post partum hemorrhage

76. Which of the following is a known cause of polyhyramnios?
   a. Intrauterine growth retardation
   b. Hypertensive disorders of pregnancy
   c. Post-dates pregnancy
   d. Diabetes mellitus

77. Following intrauterine fetal demise, onset of labor usually occurs within two to three weeks. This is believed to be due to which of the following factors?
   a. Breakdown of fetal membranes
   b. Increase in prostaglandin production
   c. Lack of stimulation of mechanoreceptors in the uterus
   d. Cessation of placental function

78. Which of the following is a risk of expectant management of intrauterine fetal demise?
   a. Hemorrhage
   b. Collapse of the fetal skull
   c. Disseminated intravascular coagulation (DIC)
   d. Infection

DATA FOR ITEM 79

A woman has experienced a fetal demise at 34 weeks gestation. She asks you to explain the most likely reason for the death.

79. Which of the following is the MOST appropriate response to this question?
   a. Fetal demise is usually caused by genetic abnormalities.
   b. Cord accidents are the most common cause of fetal demise at advanced gestational ages.
   c. You will have to wait for the autopsy report, which can take up to three months, to provide her with a diagnosis of the cause of death.
   d. Even after a thorough autopsy, most intrauterine deaths have no known cause.

80. In the absence of a baseline blood pressure, which of the following blood pressures would be considered hypertension?
   a. 130/80
   b. 135/88
   c. 128/90
   d. 138/78

81. Which of the following is an accurate definition of proteinuria?
   a. Protein in the urine in excess of 1 g/L
   b. Protein in the urine in excess of 2 g/L
   c. Protein in the urine in excess of 3 g/L
   d. Protein in the urine in excess of 4 g/L

82. Which of the following does NOT predispose a woman to develop preeclampsia?
   a. Trophoblastic disease
   b. Maternal age greater than 35
   c. Obesity
   d. Multiple pregnancy

83. Which of the following is NOT part of the classical clinical triad of symptoms associated with preeclampsia?
    a. Hypertension
    b. Hyperreflexia
    c. Proteinuria
    d. Edema

84. Which of the following is NOT a classical clinical sign of HELLP syndrome?
    a. Hypertension
    b. Hemolysis
    c. Elevated liver enzymes
    d. Low platelets

85. If a woman develops preeclampsia before 36 weeks gestation, the midwife should monitor for the development of which of the following associated conditions?
    a. Hyperemesis gravidarium
    b. Intrauterine growth retardation
    c. Preterm labor
    d. Sickle cell disease

86. Eclamptic seizures are usually which of the following type of seizures?
    a. Tonic-clonic
    b. Focal
    c. Grand mal
    d. Petit mal

87. When are eclamptic seizures MOST likely to occur?
    a. In the first trimester
    b. In the second trimester
    c. In the third trimester and in labor
    d. During the postpartum period

DATA FOR ITEMS 88–89

HG is a 18 year-old G1P0 with preeclampsia. You have admitted her to the hospital to initiate magnesium sulfate therapy, but she starts seizing before you can start an IV.

88. What is the MOST appropriate action at this time?
    a. Call for help, notify the physician, and try to stop the seizure with phenobarbital
    b. Call for help, notify the physician, and try to stop the seizure with magnesium sulfate
    c. Call for help, notify the physician, observe the seizure but do not try to stop it
    d. Call for help, notify the physician, observe the seizure and restrain her arms and legs to avoid injury

89. Which of the following is the top priority following the seizure?
    a. Administer oxygen by facemask since that woman had no respirations during the seizure
    b. Maintain a patent airway
    c. Evaluate fetal status
    d. Examine the woman for injury

90. Which of the following is the cardinal sign of placenta previa?
    a. Painless bleeding that is usually sudden in onset
    b. Painful bleeding that is usually sudden in onset
    c. Painless bleeding with a board-like abdomen
    d. Painful bleeding with a board-like abdomen

91. Which of the following is the MOST appropriate way to confirm a diagnosis of placenta previa?
   a. Through a careful vaginal examination in a double-setup setting
   b. Through visual confirmation with a speculum examination
   c. Through visual confirmation with an ultrasound examination
   d. Through associated symptoms like fetal malpresentation and an unengaged presenting part at term

DATA FOR ITEMS 92–93

HG, a 29-year-old G4P2102, presents with vaginal bleeding at 28 weeks gestation. She is not having uterine contractions. Ultrasound examination reveals that she has a total placenta previa. Her prenatal course has been unremarkable. She had one previous cesarean section for fetal distress and two successful vaginal births after the cesarean section (VBAC's).

92. Which of the following is the MOST appropriate management plan for HG at this time?
   a. Admit to the hospital for emergency cesarean section
   b. Admit to the hospital for tocolytic therapy
   c. Admit to the hospital for maternal blood studies and fetal assessment
   d. Admit to the hospital for tocolysis and corticosteroid therapy

93. HG is at increased risk for which of the following complications?
   a. Preeclampsia
   b. Endometritis
   c. Placenta accreta
   d. Cord prolapse

94. Which of the following is the MOST appropriate management for abruptio placenta in a woman at 34 weeks gestation?
   a. Discharge to home if woman and fetus are stable
   b. Corticosteroid treatment and delivery 24 hours after steroid therapy
   c. Immediate delivery either vaginally or by cesarean section
   d. Emergency cesarean section once lung maturity has been ascertained

95. Which of the following is the MOST common cause for size-greater-than-dates?
   a. Large fetus
   b. Breech presentation
   c. Multiple gestation
   d. Polyhydramnios

96. Which of the following is NOT a cause of size-greater-than-dates?
   a. Gestational diabetes
   b. Myomata
   c. Transverse lie
   d. Trophoblastic disease

97. Which of the following MOST accurately describes asymmetrical intrauterine growth retardation (IUGR)?
   a. Decreased head circumference with normal weight and body length
   b. Decreased head circumference, decreased weight, but normal body length
   c. Normal head circumference and normal weight, but decreased body length
   d. Normal head circumference with decreased weight and decreased body length

98. Which of the following series of findings is MOST likely to be indicative of intrauterine growth retardation (IUGR)?
   a. A woman with average body mass index (BMI) and low weight gain whose fundal height has been consistently 2 centimeters lower than estimated gestational age
   b. A woman with average body mass index (BMI) and adequate weight gain who had size consistent with dates through week 24 and 1.5 centimeter total increase in fundal height in weeks 24 through 28
   c. A woman with low body mass index (BMI) and appropriate weight gain whose fundal height has been consistently 2 centimeters lower than estimated gestational age
   d. A woman with low body mass index (BMI) and average weight gain who had a fundal height of 27 cm at 28 weeks and has had a 4 centimeter increase in fundal height in 5 weeks

99. Which of the following would be MOST helpful in confirming a clinical suspicion of intrauterine growth retardation (IUGR)?
   a. Two ultrasound measurement of biparietal diameter at least four weeks apart
   b. Two ultrasound measurements of head-abdomen ratio at least two weeks apart
   c. Two ultrasound measurements of abdominal circumference at least four weeks apart
   d. Two ultrasound measurements of head circumference at least two weeks apart

100. Which of the following is associated with severe fetal growth impairment?
   a. Preterm labor
   b. Pregnancy-induced hypertension
   c. Head-abdomen circumference greater than 1:1
   d. Oligohydramnios

101. Which of the following birthweights is the established norm in the United States for a diagnosis of large-for-gestational age (LGA)?
   a. 3800 grams
   b. 4000 grams
   c. 4200 grams
   d. 4500 grams

102. Which of the following statements about postmaturity syndrome is TRUE?
   a. It occurs in a majority of postdates pregnancies.
   b. It can happen independently of a postdate pregnancy.
   c. It usually results in a large-for-gestational age infant.
   d. It is most likely caused by decreasing uteroplacental function.

103. What percentage of pregnancies that are labeled postdates are actually postdates pregnancies?
   a. Approximately 10%
   b. Approximately 30%
   c. Approximately 50%
   d. Approximately 60%

104. When should you initiate and how often should you conduct nonstress testing (NST) in a postdates pregnancy when there are normal fetal movement counts (FMC)?
   a. Initiate at 40 weeks and once a week thereafter
   b. Initiate at 40 weeks and twice weekly thereafter
   c. Initiate at 41–42 weeks and once a week thereafter
   d. Initiate at 41–42 weeks and twice weekly thereafter

Chapter 10 Answer Key

Antepartal Complications

1. c p. 328	**27.** b p. 340	**53.** b p. 349	**79.** d p. 359
2. d p. 328	**28.** b p. 340	**54.** d p. 349	**80.** c p. 360
3. a p. 328	**29.** c p. 340	**55.** c p. 348	**81.** a p. 360
4. b p. 329	**30.** a p. 341	**56.** c p. 349	**82.** c p. 360
5. c p. 329	**31.** a p. 341	**57.** b p. 350	**83.** b p. 361
6. c p. 327	**32.** a p. 341	**58.** d p. 351	**84.** a p. 363
7. b p. 329	**33.** d p. 342	**59.** a p. 351	**85.** b p. 363
8. c p. 330	**34.** d p. 342	**60.** c p. 352	**86.** a p. 363
9. d p. 331	**35.** a p. 343	**61.** b p. 353	**87.** c p. 363
10. d p. 331	**36.** c p. 343	**62.** b p. 353	**88.** c p. 363–364
11. b p. 331	**37.** b p. 343	**63.** a p. 353	**89.** b p. 364
12. d p. 331	**38.** b p. 344	**64.** d p. 354	**90.** a p. 365
13. d p. 331	**39.** c p. 344	**65.** d p. 353	**91.** c p. 365
14. c p. 331	**40.** b p. 344	**66.** b p. 354	**92.** c p. 365
15. c p. 331	**41.** b p. 344	**67.** d p. 354–355	**93.** c p. 366
16. d p. 335	**42.** d p. 344	**68.** a p. 355–356	**94.** c p. 367
17. c p. 335	**43.** c p. 345	**69.** a p. 356	**95.** a p. 368–369
18. b p. 336	**44.** b p. 346	**70.** d p. 357	**96.** c p. 369
19. b p. 336	**45.** a p. 345	**71.** b p. 357	**97.** d p. 370
20. c p. 336–337	**46.** c p. 346	**72.** b p. 357	**98.** b p. 370
21. a p. 337	**47.** b p. 346	**73.** c p. 358	**99.** c p. 370
22. d p. 338	**48.** a p. 346	**74.** b p. 358	**100.** d p. 371
23. c p. 337	**49.** a p. 320	**75.** b p. 357	**101.** b p. 372
24. b p. 338	**50.** a p. 347	**76.** d p. 357	**102.** d p. 373
25. a p. 338	**51.** b p. 348	**77.** d p. 359	**103.** b p. 374
26. b p. 339	**52.** d p. 349	**78.** c p. 359	**104.** d p. 374

PART IV: INTRAPARTUM CARE

PART IV

Chapter 11 Outline
False and Early Labor and The Normal First Stage of Labor

I.   **Stages of Labor**

     A. Diagnosis/Definitions

     B. Limits of normal

     C. Friedman Labor Curve

II.   **Recognizing/Assessing Signs and Symptoms of Impending Labor**

     A. Lightening

     B. Cervical changes/Cervical ripening
        Bishop Score

     C. Rupture of membranes

     D. Bloody show

     E. Energy spurt

     F. Gastrointestinal upsets

III.   **Diagnosis of Labor**

     A. Contractions—assessment and parameters of normal

        1. Frequency

        2. Duration

        3. Intensity

        4. Gradient pattern

        5. Montevideo units

     B. Cervical changes—assessment and parameters of normal

        1. Effacement

        2. Dilation

        3. Position

     C. Station—assessment and parameters of normal

     D. Rupture of membranes—diagnosis

IV.   **Differentiating False/Prodromal Labor vs. Early/Latent Labor vs. Active Labor**

     A. Contractions

        1. onset

        2. duration

        3. frequency

        4. alleviating or aggravating factors

     B. Cervical dilation

V.   Management of False/Prodromal Labor and Early/Latent Labor

A. Comfort measures

B. Medications
1. type/classification
2. dose
3. route
4. frequency
5. contraindications
6. side effects

C. Parameters of normal

VI.   Initial Evaluation of the Woman and Fetus in Labor

A. Identifying Information
1. Name
2. Age
3. Race
4. Gravity and Parity
5. Last menstrual period (LMP)
6. Estimated date of delivery (EDD)
7. Estimated gestational age (EGA)

B. Obstetrical History
1. History of present labor
   a. Contractions—frequency, duration, onset, intensity
   b. Bloody show/Mucus plug
   c. Rupture of membranes—onset, timing in relation to start of contractions, presence of blood or meconium
   d. Vaginal bleeding—spotting vs. frank bleeding
   e. Fetal movement
   f. Most recent meal
   g. Hydration status
2. History of present pregnancy
   a. Date that she started receiving prenatal care
   b. Number of prenatal visits
   c. Location of prenatal care
   d. Antepartal complications
   e. Medical complications
   f. Drugs and medications taken during pregnancy
   g. Antepartal fetal testing (ultrasound, BPP, amniocentesis)
3. Past obstetrical history
   a. Number of past pregnancies
   b. Dates of past pregnancies/deliveries
   c. Duration of past pregnancies
   d. Outcome of past pregnancies (term delivery, preterm delivery, spontaneous or induced abortions, ectopic pregnancies)

      e. Complications of last pregnancies (including preterm labor and preterm birth)

      f. Duration of past labors

      g. Complications of last labors

C. Past Medical and Surgical History (including any known allergies to medications)

    1. Family and social history (including any substance abuse during pregnancy)

    2. Review of systems

D. Physical Examination

    1. Vital signs

    2. Head, ears, eyes, nose, throat (HEENT)

    3. Chest (including lung and heart auscultations)

    4. Abdominal/Leopold's Maneuvers

      a. Contraction pattern/Contraction intensity

      b. Uterine size

      c. Estimated fetal weight

      d. Position of fetus (lie, presentation, position, variety)

      e. Fetal movements

      f. Engagement

    5. Extremities

      a. Edema

      b. Deep tendon reflexes

E. Pelvic Examination

    1. Sterile speculum exam if necessary to confirm rupture of membranes

    2. Sterile vaginal exam

      a. Status of membranes

      b. Cervical effacement, dilation, position

      c. Fetal station and position (lie, presentation, position, variety)

      d. Presence of molding or caput succedaneum

      e. Presence of synclitism/asyclitism

      f. Clinical pelvimetry/Evaluation of vaginal and perineal muscle tone

F. Laboratory Tests

    1. Review prenatal laboratory test results

    2. Obtain/order CBC, RPR, blood type and cross-match, and urinalysis and other tests as indicated or required by law

G. Fetal Heart Rate

    1. Baseline

    2. Variability

    3. Presence of accelerations

    4. Presence of decelerations

VII. First Stage of Labor

A. Definition/Latent vs. Active Stage

B. Transition

    1. Definition

    2. Signs and symptoms of transition

C. Parameters of Normal/Friedman Curve

VIII. Assessment of Maternal Progress in First Stage of Labor

A. Cervical Status

    1. Effacement

    2. Dilatation

    3. Station

    4. Friedman Curve

    5. Frequency/Indications for cervical assessment/vaginal examinations

B. Contraction Patterns/Monitoring of Contractions in Labor

    1. Parameters of Normal

        a. Baseline

        b. Frequency

        c. Intensity

        d. Duration

    2. Methods of Evaluation

        a. Palpation

        b. Tocometer

        c. Intrauterine Pressure Catheter (IUPC)

            i. Indications/Contraindications

            ii. Interpretation and management of IUPC strip

            iii. Montevideo units (calculate and know significance of)

    3. Dysfunctional Contractions Patterns (Discussed further in Chapter 13)

C. Vital Signs

    Frequency

D. Bladder Status

E. Hydration Status

F. General Condition

IX. Maternal Physiological Changes During Labor

A. Blood pressure

B. Metabolism

C. Temperature

D. Heart Rate/Pulse

E. Respiratory Rate/Respirations

F. Renal function

G. Gastrointestinal function

H. Hematologic status (hemoglobin/hematocrit, platelets, WBC's, blood sugar, coagulation factors, etc.)

X. Fetal "Position"

A. Lie

B. Presentation

C. Position

D. Variety

E. Attitude

F. Synclitism

G. Asynclitism (anterior vs. posterior)

H. Molding and Caput Succedaneum

Know the following for each of the above:
   1. Definition
   2. Diagnosis
   3. Significance/Management

XI. The Fetal Skull

Know and be able to identify the following fetal skull landmarks:

A. Bones
   1. frontal
   2. parietal
   3. occipital

B. Sutures
   1. frontal
   2. sagittal
   3. coronal
   4. lamboid

C. Fontanels
   1. anterior
   2. posterior

D. Diameters
   1. biparietal
   2. suboccipitobregmatic
   3. occipitofrontal
   4. occipitomental
   5. submentalbregmatic

XII. Fetal Heart Tones/Evaluation of Fetus in Labor

A. Baseline fetal heart rate
   1. Parameters of normal
   2. Bradycardia (moderate vs. marked)
   3. Tachycardia (moderate vs. marked)

B. Variability (short-term vs. long-term variability)
Parameters of normal

C. Periodic fetal heart rate changes

    1. Parameters of normal

    2. Accelerations

    3. Early decelerations

    4. Other decelerations (outlined in detail in Chapter 13)

D. Methods of evaluation

    1. Fetoscope

    2. Ultrasound

    3. External fetal monitoring

        a. Continuous

            i. Indications

            ii. Interpretation of fetal monitor strips

            iii. Parameters of normal

        b. Intermittent (ACOG guidelines for Intermittent Auscultation)

            i. Indications/Contraindications

            ii. Frequency

            iii. Parameters of normal

        c. Internal fetal monitoring

            i. Indications/Contraindications

            ii. Interpretation of fetal monitor strips

            iii. Parameters of normal

        d. Fetal scalp pH

            i. Indications

            ii. Interpretation and management of results

            iii. Parameters of normal

E. Evaluation for caput succedaneum and/or molding

F. Fetal indications for vaginal examinations

XIII. Management of First Stage of Labor

A. Maternal and Fetal Evaluation (See above)

B. Pain Management

    1. Non-pharmacological interventions

        a. Indications/contraindications

        b. Timing

        c. Assessment of effectiveness

    2. Pharmacological interventions (analgesia)

        a. Type

        b. Indications/contraindications

        c. Timing (appropriate stage of labor)

        d. Dose

        e. Route

        f. Frequency

        g. Side effects/potential complications

> **3.** Pharmacological interventions (anesthesia)
>> **a.** Epidural/Pudendal Block/Local
>>> **i.** Timing (appropriate stage of labor)
>>> **ii.** Indications/Contraindications
>>> **iii.** Technique/Medication/Dose (for Pudendal and Local)
>>> **iv.** Side effects/potential complications

C. Rupture of Membranes
> **1.** Confirmation of spontaneous rupture of membranes (SROM)
> **2.** Artificial rupture of membranes (AROM)/Amniotomy
>> **a.** Indications/contraindications
>> **b.** Technique
>> **c.** Side effects/potential complications

D. Maternal Support/Comfort Measures
> **1.** Ambulation/position changes
> **2.** Relaxation techniques/Breathing techniques
> **3.** Temperature regulation
> **4.** Massage/Use of heat and cold/Abdominal rub/Effleurage

E. Management of Anterior Cervical Lip

F. Additional Issues
> **1.** Significant others in the labor room
> **2.** Nutrition and hydration in labor
> **3.** Enemas
> **4.** Perineal Shaves/Perineal Preps
> **5.** Intravenous fluids/Heparin or Saline locks
> **6.** Urinary catheterization

XIV. Vaginal Birth After Cesarean Section (VBAC)

A. Indications/Contraindications (selection of candidates for VBAC)

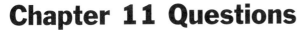

Chapter 11 Questions
False and Early Labor and the Normal First Stage of Labor

1. Which of the following statements about lightening is TRUE?
  a. It usually occurs before labor in multigravidas but not in primigravidas.
  b. It can be used to predict the onset of labor.
  c. It will lower fundal height to a position similar to that of the eighth month of pregnancy.
  d. It will relieve shortness of breath, leg cramps, and dependent edema.

2. When in pregnancy do Braxton-Hicks contractions begin?
  a. At approximately 6 weeks gestation
  b. At approximately 10 weeks gestation
  c. At approximately 16 weeks gestation
  d. At approximately 20 weeks gestation

3. What percentage of women at or near term will start labor spontaneously within 24 hours of premature rupture of membranes?
  a. Approximately 20%
  b. Approximately 40%
  c. Approximately 60%
  d. Approximately 80%

4. Which of the following BEST describes the cervix of the average primigravida on the verge of true labor?
  a. 50 to 100 percent effaced with a fingertip to 1 centimeter dilation
  b. 50 to 60 percent effaced with 2 to 3 centimeters dilation
  c. Little or no effacement with a fingertip to 1 centimeter dilation
  d. Little or no effacement with 1 to 2 centimeters or more dilation

5. Which of the following women is NOT a good candidate for an out-of hospital birth?
  a. A grand multipara
  b. A primigravida with a large fetus
  c. A multipara with a breech presentation
  d. A primigravida older than 35 years of age

6. Which of the following is the BEST description of how uterine contractions differentiate the uterus into two segments?
  a. The upper zone of the uterus shortens and thickens, while the lower zone lengthens and thins.
  b. The upper zone of the uterus lengthens and thickens, while the lower zone shortens and thins.
  c. The upper zone of the uterus shortens and thins, while the lower segment lengthens and thickens.
  d. The upper zone of the uterus remains fixed in length, while the lower segment shortens and thins.

7. Which of the following indicators BEST enables a midwife to diagnose the onset of true labor?
  a. The onset of a regular contraction pattern
  b. The rupture of membranes
  c. The expulsion of the mucus plug
  d. Progressive cervical effacement and dilation

8. Which of the following is the BEST definition of fetal engagement?

   a. When the widest diameter of the fetal presenting part is at zero station
   b. When the lowermost part of the fetal presenting part has passed through the pelvic inlet
   c. When the lowermost part of the fetal presenting part is at zero station
   d. When the widest diameter of the fetal presenting part has passed through the pelvic inlet

9. Which of the following landmarks of the fetal head would you use to determine station in a well-flexed, cephalic presentation?

   a. The parietal prominences
   b. The occipital bone
   c. The sagittal suture
   d. The caput

10. Which of the following is NOT a characteristic of true labor contractions?

   a. They are regular.
   b. They increase in frequency, duration, and intensity.
   c. They radiate from the fundus to the back.
   d. They are relieved by walking.

11. Which of the following findings would be LEAST likely to give a false positive result when confirming rupture of membranes?

   a. A positive nitrazine test
   b. A positive ferning test
   c. Being unable to visualize or feel the membranes bulging over the presenting part
   d. Visualizing amniotic fluid escaping from the cervical os

DATA FOR ITEMS 12–15

TR is a 22 year-old G1P0 at 39 weeks gestation with an unremarkable prenatal course. She calls you at 10 p.m. because she has been having contractions since 11 a.m. and is unable to sleep now and is exhausted. She has had no signs of rupture of membranes and has no bleeding. Her contractions have been every 10 to 30 minutes, lasting 20 to 30 seconds. She states that the contractions have not become more intense or changed in character but that she is uncomfortable especially when lying or sitting down and feels better when she is ambulating. She reports normal fetal movement.

12. You suspect that TR is experiencing which of the following?

   a. False labor
   b. Early latent phase of labor
   c. Late latent phase of labor
   d. Deceleration phase of labor

13. What is your BEST management option at this time?

   a. Have TR meet you at your office so that you can examine her
   b. Have TR meet you at the hospital so that you can examine her
   c. Suggest to TR that she take a warm bath and have a hot drink with sugar and to call you back if she is unable to sleep
   d. Suggest to TR that she walk around the house to try to establish a more regular contraction pattern

ADDITIONAL DATA FOR ITEMS 14–15

At 2:00 in the morning, you examine TR and she is 90% effaced and 2 centimeters dilated. Her contractions are now of moderate intensity, occurring every 7 to 10 minutes, and lasting 20 to 40 seconds. She has had no sleep, is extremely tired, and is becoming frustrated. The fetus has a cephalic presentation and is at –1 station. Fetal heart rate is in the 130's with no decelerations.

14. TR is MOST likely experiencing which of the following?
 a. False labor
 b. Latent phase of labor
 c. Early active phase of labor
 d. Phase of maximum slope of labor

15. Which is the BEST management option in the care of TR at this point?
 a. Admit her to the hospital and encourage her to ambulate
 b. Admit her to the hospital and give her some morphine
 c. Send her home and have her ambulate at home
 d. Send her home with some sedatives and encourage her to rest

16. During what stage of labor does the majority of progressive descent of the fetal presenting part occur?
 a. During the latent phase
 b. During the phase of maximum slope
 c. During the deceleration phase and during second stage
 d. During second stage

17. Which of the following signs and symptoms of the transitional phase is NOT a traditional sign of impending second stage?
 a. Uncontrollable desire to bear down
 b. Severe low backache
 c. Expulsive grunt upon exhalation
 d. Rupture of membranes

18. Which of the following is NOT a term used to describe the lie of the fetus?
 a. Longitudinal
 b. Transverse
 c. Vertex
 d. Oblique

■ **DATA FOR ITEMS 19–20**

On vaginal exam you feel the occiput on the right anterior portion of the maternal pelvis.

19. Which of the following is used to describe this fetus' position?
 a. RO
 b. LO
 c. OT
 d. OA

20. Which of the following is used to describe this fetus' variety?
 a. Military
 b. Flexed
 c. OT
 d. OA

21. Which of the following is the most common position, lie, presentation and variety of the fetus at the onset of labor?
 a. ROP
 b. ROT
 c. LOT
 d. LOP

22. The anterior fontanel of the fetal skull is formed by the meeting of which sutures?
    a. Frontal, sagittal, and coronal
    b. Frontal, lamboidal, and coronal
    c. Frontal, sagittal, and lamboidal
    d. Frontal and sagittal

23. The posterior fontanel is roughly the shape of which of the following?
    a. A rhomboid
    b. A diamond
    c. A triangle
    d. An oval

24. Which is the only suture on the fetal head that has the anterior fontanel at one end and the posterior fontanel at the other?
    a. Coronal suture
    b. Frontal suture
    c. Lamboidal suture
    d. Sagittal suture

■ **DATA FOR ITEM 25**

On vaginal exam you feel that the fetus is ROT and that the sagittal suture is tilted toward the maternal symphysis pubis.

25. The fetal head is said to have which of the following?
    a. Anterior asynclitism
    b. Posterior asynclitism
    c. Transverse asynclitism
    d. Synclitism

26. In normal labor, the head usually enters the pelvic inlet with a moderate degree of which of the following?
    a. Anterior asynclitism
    b. Posterior asynclitism
    c. Transverse asynclitism
    d. Synclitism

27. Which of the following terms is used to describe the change in the shape of the fetal head as a result of the overriding of the fetal skull bones?
    a. Asynclitism
    b. Molding
    c. Caput
    d. Cephalhematoma

28. What is the term used to describe changes in fetal heart rate that are associated with uterine contractions?
    a. Accelerations
    b. Decelerations
    c. Periodic changes
    d. Variability

29. Which of the following is considered the normal range for fetal heart rate?
    a. 100 to 160 beats per minute
    b. 110 to 160 beats per minute
    c. 120 to 160 beats per minute
    d. 130 to 160 beats per minute

30. Which of the following fetal heart rates is considered the cut-off for marked tachycardia?
    a. Above 170 beats per minute
    b. Above 180 beats per minute
    c. Above 190 beats per minute
    d. Above 200 beats per minute

31. Which is the BEST method for the midwife to intermittently listen to fetal heart tones during labor?
    a. Start listening at the beginning of a contraction through to the beginning of the next contraction
    b. Wait 30 seconds after a contraction, start listening and then listen until the beginning of the next contraction
    c. Start listening midway between two contractions and continue listening through the next contraction and until the beginning of the following contraction
    d. Start listening midway between two contractions and continue listening through the next contraction to the midpoint between it and the following contraction

32. Which of the following is NOT a risk of rupture of membranes?
    a. Formation of caput succedaneum
    b. Head trauma leading to brain damage
    c. Fetal scalp abscess
    d. Cord prolapse

33. Which of the following methods of fetal heart evaluation provides the most reliable, comprehensive data?
    a. Intermittent auscultation with a Doptone or fetoscope
    b. Continuous monitoring with an external monitor
    c. Auscultated acceleration test with Doptone or fetoscope
    d. Continuous monitoring with an internal monitor

34. Which of the following is considered the critical level of fetal scalp pH at which immediate delivery becomes necessary?
    a. Second reading of a pH < 7.30
    b. Second reading of a pH < 7.25
    c. Second reading of a pH < 7.20
    d. Second reading of a pH < 7.10

35. Which of the following represents a NORMAL rise of blood pressure during contractions for a woman in labor?
    a. A systolic rise of 5–10 mm Hg and a diastolic rise of 0–5 mm Hg
    b. A systolic rise of 10–20 mm Hg and a diastolic rise of 5–10 mm Hg
    c. A systolic rise of 15–25 mm Hg and a diastolic rise of 5–15 mm Hg
    d. A systolic rise of 25–30 mm Hg and a diastolic rise of 10–20 mm Hg

36. Which of the following is the reasoning commonly used to keep women from eating any solids during labor?
    a. It will reduce the chances of vomiting and aspiration during transition and second stage of labor.
    b. It will reduce the chances of aspiration in the event of need for a cesarean section.
    c. Is will reduce the chances of aspiration in the event of need for general anesthesia.
    d. It will increase the chances of a sterile field for delivery.

37. Which of the following women does NOT need to have an IV during her labor?

  a. A G6P4104 in normal labor
  b. A G2P1001 with an estimated fetal weight of 9 1/2 pounds
  c. A G4P4004 at 42 weeks gestation in spontaneous labor
  d. A G2P0010 expecting twins

38. Which of the following maternal positions will be MOST helpful in facilitating the long arc rotation of a fetus in ROP?

  a. Knee-chest position
  b. Semi-recumbent position
  c. Left-lateral position
  d. Right-lateral position

■ **DATA FOR ITEM 39**

DS is a 26-year-old G1P0 at 38 weeks gestation. She has come into your office at noon for a labor check. Her contractions started about 10 hours earlier at which point they were approximately 15 minutes apart and lasting approximately 40 seconds. Now she is having contractions about every 10 minutes lasting about 45 to 60 seconds. She is uncomfortable with the contractions but is relaxed and coping well. She has not had any bleeding or rupture of membranes. Your exam reveals that she is 100% effaced and at 2 centimeters dilation. The fetal head is at 0 station. Fetal heart rate is in the 140's with no decelerations.

39. What is your BEST management plan for DS at this time?

  a. Admit her to the hospital with a plan to ambulate and take a warm shower
  b. Admit her to the hospital with a plan to start pitocin to establish effective contraction pattern
  c. Send her home with the expectation that active labor will set in later during the day
  d. Send her home with some sedatives so she can get some rest

■ **DATA FOR ITEM 40**

SF, a 28-year-old G3P2002, comes to the hospital in advanced labor. She is 100% effaced and 7 centimeters dilated and the fetal head is at +2 station. Her membranes are ruptured. You expect that delivery will take place in the next three or four hours. SF does not want an epidural, but does want some medication to alleviate the pain of contractions. The fetal heart rate is 140 and there are occasional variable decelerations.

40. Which of the following is your BEST pain management plan for SF?

  a. Offer 2 mg of Stadol IM
  b. Offer 15 mg of Morphine IM
  c. Offer 100 mg Seconal po
  d. Offer only non-pharmacologic methods so that the newborn will not suffer respiratory depression

41. How often should the fetal heart rate and pattern be evaluated through auscultation during a normal, active, first stage of labor?

  a. Every 15 minutes
  b. Every 20 minutes
  c. Every 30 minutes
  d. Every 60 minutes

42. Which of the following is NOT an indication for a vaginal exam in a normal, progressive labor?

  a. On admission, to establish a baseline
  b. Before deciding on kind, amount, and route of medication
  c. Following a prolonged period of ambulation or prolonged period in the shower
  d. To verify complete dilation

43. Which of the following describes the technique of controlled relaxation?

    a. Keeping one muscle group relaxed while another muscle group is contracted

    b. Taking a deep breath and letting it out in a heavy sigh after a contraction

    c. Using mental imagery to distract thoughts from painful stimuli

    d. Deliberately tightening a single muscle group as tight as possible and then letting it go as limp as possible and then repeating exercise with a different muscle group

DATA FOR ITEM 44

You are a new midwife at a large, tertiary, teaching hospital. One of your clients is in second stage and one of the residents approaches you and asks you to obtain consent from your client for two medical students to observe the birth. The resident asked the woman for permission earlier in labor, but was denied and so the resident wants you to intervene.

44. What is the MOST appropriate course of action at this point?

    a. Tell the resident that as long as they remain quiet and out of the way, the students can observe the birth.

    b. Explain to your client the nature of a teaching hospital and attempt to convince her to allow the students in for the birth.

    c. Tell the resident that since the woman is already pushing, it is not an appropriate time to intervene, but that the students can come in for the birth of your other client who is still in first stage.

    d. Tell the resident that since the patient already declined consent it is inappropriate for you to intervene, particularly at this stage in labor.

45. Which of the following procedures can NOT be performed in an out-of-hospital birth setting?

    a. Artificial rupture of membranes

    b. Newborn resuscitation

    c. Administration of antibiotics as prophylaxis for GBS

    d. Pitocin augmentation

Chapter 11 Answer Key
False and Early Labor and the First Stage of Labor

1. *c* p. 381

2. *a* p. 382

3. *d* p. 382

4. *a* p. 385

5. *c* p. 535

6. *a* p. 384–385

7. *d* p. 385

8. *d* p. 386

9. *b* p. 386

10. *d* p. 387

11. *d* p. 390

12. *a* p. 382, 387, 395–396

13. *c* p. 391–392

14. *b* p. 385–386, 396

15. *d* p. 391–392

16. *c* p. 396

17. *b* p. 397

18. *c* p. 398–399

19. *a* p. 399

20. *d* p. 399

21. *c* p. 399

22. *a* p. 401

23. *c* p. 401

24. *d* p. 400

25. *b* p. 401

26. *b* p. 401

27. *b* p. 402

28. *c* p. 402

29. *c* p. 402

30. *b* p. 403

31. *d* p. 403

32. *c* p. 404–405

33. *d* p. 404

34. *c* p. 405

35. *b* p. 406

36. *c* p. 410

37. *c* p. 411

38. *d* p. 412

39. *c* p. 391–392

40. *a* p. 413–414

41. *c* p. 417

42. *c* p. 419

43. *a* p. 424

44. *d* p. 426

45. *d* p. 536

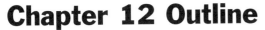

Chapter 12 Outline

The Normal Second Stage of Labor

I. **Second Stage of Labor**

    A. Definition

    B. Parameters of normal/Friedman Curve

II. **Maternal and Fetal Assessment (Discussed further in Chapter 9)**

    A. Maternal pushing effort

        Physiological vs. directed pushing effort

    B. Perineal integrity/Need for an episiotomy

III. **Mechanisms of Labor**

    Be able to describe the eight basic positional movements including degree rotation for the various positions of the fetus as it enters labor. (e.g. Be able to describe the positional movements for a fetus that starts labor in LOP and is born in OA.)

    A. Engagement

    B. Descent

    C. Flexion

    D. Internal rotation _____ to the _____ position (short vs. long arc rotation)

    E. Birth (by extension or by flexion and extension)

    F. Restitution 45° to the _____ position

    G. External rotation 45° to the _____ position

    H. Birth of the shoulders

IV. **Maternal Positions for Delivery**

V. **Preparation for Delivery**

    A. Notification of nursing/back-up staff

    B. Preparation of newborn resuscitation equipment/supplies

    C. Surgical scrub/Gowning/Gloving

    D. Universal precautions

    E. Preparation of sterile instruments/equipment (clamps, scissors, suction bulb)

    F. Positioning and draping of woman

VI.   Hand Maneuvers

A. Occiput anterior
1. Lithotomy
2. Semi-recumbent
3. Side-lying/Other maternal positions

B. Occiput posterior
1. Lithotomy
2. Semi-recumbent
3. Side-lying/Other maternal positions

C. Breech/Other presentations

D. Ritgen maneuver/Modified Ritgen maneuver

VII.   Episiotomy

A. Timing/Technique (Including local anesthetic infiltration)
1. Midline
2. Mediolateral

B. Indications
1. Midline
2. Mediolateral

VIII.   Management of Nuchal Cord/Nuchal Arm

IX.   Cutting and Clamping of the Umbilical Cord

A. Immediate vs. delayed

X.   Immediate Care/Assessment of Newborn

A. Suctioning/Maintaining patent airway

B. Thermoregulation

C. Resuscitation (Discussed further in Chapter 18)

D. Apgar scores

E. Immediate exam/assessment of newborn (Discussed further in Chapter 19)

Chapter 12 Questions
The Normal Second Stage of Labor

1. Second stage is known as which of the following?
   a. Deceleration phase
   b. Pushing stage
   c. Expulsion stage
   d. Bearing-down phase

2. According to Friedman, what is the average length of second stage for primigravidas?
   a. 30 minutes
   b. 60 minutes
   c. 90 minutes
   d. 120 minutes

DATA FOR ITEM 3

A woman who is a G3P2002 is in active labor and turns to you and cries, "The baby is coming!" You checked the woman 15 minutes ago and she was 8 centimeters dilated and the fetal head was at 0 station.

3. What is your BEST response to her comment?
   a. Tell her that you will check her dilation after the next contraction is over
   b. Tell her that what she is feeling is most likely due to progressive descent of the fetal head
   c. Ask her to start panting respirations and while keeping your eyes on the perineum, put on your gloves
   d. Ask her not to push because, if she is not fully dilated, she might injure her cervix

DATA FOR ITEM 4–5

The uterine contractions of a woman who has just completed cervical dilation space out and are no longer as intense as they were previously. This pattern has been present for approximately 20 minutes and the woman feels no urge to push. The woman's labor progress has been normal to this point.

4. Which of the following is the BEST management option at this time?
   a. Initiate Pitocin augmentation to reestablish an effective contraction pattern
   b. Insert an intra-uterine pressure catheter to determine whether the contractions are adequate to effect delivery
   c. Continue with a watchful waiting approach
   d. Prepare for a probable instrumental delivery or cesarean section

ADDITIONAL DATA FOR ITEM 5

Another hour passes and the woman's contractions have increased some in frequency and intensity. The contractions are every 4–5 minutes and lasting approximately 45–60 seconds. The fetal head is at +1 station and has not changed in the last hour. You can feel that the sagittal suture is in a transverse diameter. The pressure of the contractions is of 20–30mm Hg as determined by an intrauterine pressure catheter.

5. Which of the following is the BEST management option at this time?
   a. Initiate Pitocin augmentation to reestablish an effective contraction pattern
   b. Perform an amniotomy
   c. Continue with a watchful waiting approach
   d. Prepare for a probable instrumental delivery or cesarean section

6. Which of the following cephalic presentations means that the LARGEST diameter of the fetal head will be presenting?
   a. Vertex
   b. Military
   c. Brow
   d. Face

7. Which of the following mechanisms of labor occurs throughout labor?
   a. Engagement
   b. Descent
   c. Flexion
   d. Internal rotation

8. Birth of the head occurs through which of the following mechanisms for an occiput-anterior delivery?
   a. Flexion
   b. Extension
   c. Flexion then extension
   d. Extension then flexion

9. External rotation accomplishes which of the following in a birth with cephalic presentation?
   a. Substitutes the larger fetal head diameter for the smaller suboccipitobregmatic diameter
   b. Untwists the fetal neck and brings the head into a right angle with the shoulders
   c. Brings the anteroposterior diameter of the fetal head into alignment with the anteroposterior diameter of the maternal pelvis
   d. Brings the bisacromial diameter of the fetus into alignment with the anteroposterior diameter of the pelvic outlet

10. Internal rotation accomplishes which of the following in a birth with cephalic presentation?
    a. Substitutes a larger fetal head diameter for the smaller suboccipitobregmatic diameter
    b. Untwists the fetal neck and brings the head into a right angle with the shoulders
    c. Brings the anteroposterior diameter of the fetal head into alignment with the anteroposterior diameter of the maternal pelvis
    d. Brings the bisacromial diameter of the fetus into alignment with the anteroposterior diameter of the pelvic outlet

11. If engagement took place in ROP position, how many degrees does the fetal head rotate during internal rotation for an occiput-anterior delivery?
    a. 45
    b. 90
    c. 135
    d. 180

DATA FOR ITEMS 12–14

Assume engagement in ROT position and birth in the OA position.

12. How many degrees does the fetal head rotate during internal rotation ?
    a. 45°
    b. 90°
    c. 135°
    d. 180°

13. The head will restitute to which of the following positions?
    a. ROA
    b. ROT
    c. ROP
    d. OA

14. External rotation will bring the fetal head into which of the following positions?
   a. ROA
   b. ROT
   c. ROP
   d. OA

15. If on abdominal exam you feel the fetal back on the maternal left side and on vaginal exam you feel the sagittal suture in the right oblique diameter, what is the position of the fetus?
   a. ROA
   b. ROP
   c. LOA
   d. LOP

16. Early decelerations are believed to be caused by which of the following?
   a. Uteroplacental insufficiency
   b. Cord compression
   c. Head compression
   d. Transient fetal hypoxia

17. Which of the following physiological changes is ABNORMAL for a woman in second stage of labor?
   a. An increase in blood pressure of 20 mm Hg during contractions
   b. Tachycardia at the time of delivery
   c. Maternal temperature elevation of 2 degrees Fahrenheit
   d. Persistent, constant vomiting

18. The generally accepted frequency of blood pressure checks during second stage of labor is which of the following?
   a. Every 10 minutes
   b. Every 15 minutes
   c. Every 30 minutes
   d. Every 60 minutes

19. For which of the following is the lithotomy position for delivery contraindicated?
   a. Malpresentation
   b. Severe varicosities
   c. Multiple gestation
   d. Probable shoulder dystocia

20. Which of the following BEST describes the purpose of the Ritgen maneuver?
   a. To control the birth of the baby's head
   b. To help turn a fetus in the occiput posterior position into an occiput anterior position
   c. To help deliver a shoulder impacted under the symphysis pubis
   d. To determine whether the placenta has separated from the uterine wall

21. Which of the following is the usual concentration of lidocaine hydrochloride (Xylocaine) used for a pudendal block?
   a. 0.01%
   b. 0.1%
   c. 1%
   d. 10%

22. What is the BEST gauge to use for local infiltration of the perineal body?

    a. 20

    b. 22

    c. 24

    d. 25

23. What is the primary disadvantage of local infiltration of lidocaine for repair of an episiotomy?

    a. It requires more anesthetic than a pudendal block.

    b. It is more painful for the woman than a pudendal block.

    c. It distorts the local tissue making repair more difficult.

    d. It cannot be used for periurethral lacerations.

Chapter 12 Answer Key

The Normal Second Stage of Labor

1. *c* p. 433

2. *b* p. 433

3. *c* p. 435

4. *c* p. 433

5. *a* p. 269 PM

6. *c* p. 435

7. *b* p. 436

8. *b* p. 436

9. *d* p. 437

10. *c* p. 436

11. *c* p. 437

12. *b* p. 437

13. *a* p. 437

14. *b* p. 437

15. *c* p. 730–793

16. *c* p. 440

17. *d* p. 441

18. *b* p. 442

19. *b* p. 451

20. *a* p. 454

21. *c* p. 817

22. *b* p. 821

23. *c* p. 822

Chapter 13 Outline
Complications of the First and Second Stages of Labor

I.   Preterm Labor

A. Definition

B. Predisposing factors

C. Signs and symptoms

D. Diagnosis

E. Management

    1. Use of tocolytics

        a. Indications/contraindications

        b. Type, route, dose, frequency, side effects, potential complications

    2. Use of corticosteroids

        a. Indications/contraindications

II.   Premature Rupture of Membranes (PROM)

A. Definition

B. Predisposing factors

C. Signs and symptoms

D. Diagnosis

E. Management

    1. Group B streptococcus culture

    2. Induction vs. expectant management

    3. Signs and symptoms of chorioamnionitis

F. Management of preterm premature rupture of members (PPROM)

III.   Amnionitis and Chorioamnionitis

A. Definition

B. Predisposing factors

C. Signs and symptoms

D. Diagnosis

E. Management

    1. Antibiotic therapy

    2. Maternal/neonatal cultures

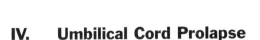

IV. Umbilical Cord Prolapse

    A. Definition (frank vs. occult)

    B. Predisposing factors

    C. Signs and symptoms

    D. Diagnosis

    E. Management

V. Cervical Ripening and Induction of Labor

    A. Indications/contraindications

    B. Bishop Scoring System

    C. Methods of cervical ripening and induction

        1. Non-pharmacologic

        2. Pharmacolgic

            a. Use of Oxytocics

                i. Indications/contraindications

                ii. Type

                iii. dose

                iv. route

                v. side effects

                vi. potential complications

        3. Uterine hyperstimulation

            a. Diagnosis

            b. Management

VI. Group Beta Streptococcus

    A. CDC Screening Protocols

    B. Intrapartum management

VII. HIV Infection

    A. Intrapartum Management

VIII. Abnormal Fetal Heart Rates and Patterns

For all of the following, know how to (visually) recognize on a fetal monitor strip:

    A. Tachycardia

        1. Definition

        2. Causes

        3. Management

    B. Bradycardia

        1. Definition

        2. Causes

        3. Management

C. Minimal or absent variability
  1. Definition
  2. Causes
  3. Management

D. Late decelerations
  1. Definition
  2. Causes
  3. Management
      a. Fetal scalp stimulation
      b. Fetal scalp blood pH sampling

E. Variable decelerations
  1. Definition
  2. Causes
  3. Management
      a. Amnioinfusion

F. Prolonged decelerations
  1. Definition
  2. Causes
  3. Management

G. Sinusoidal Pattern
  1. Definition
  2. Causes
  3. Management

H. Lambda Patterns
  1. Definition
  2. Causes
  3. Management

I. Wandering Baseline
  1. Definition
  2. Causes
  3. Management

IX.   Fetal Distress

A. Definition
  1. Hypoxemia vs. hypoxia vs. asphyxia

B. Causes

C. Signs and symptoms

D. Diagnosis

E. Management

X. Cephalopelvic Disproportion (CPD)

A. Definition

B. Predisposing factors

C. Signs and symptoms

D. Diagnosis

E. Management

XI. Deep Transverse Arrest

A. Definition

B. Predisposing factors

C. Signs and symptoms

D. Diagnosis

E. Management

XII. Uterine Dysfunction/Abnormal Labor Patterns

Hypertonic vs. Hypotonic Uterine Dysfunction

A. Prolonged Latent Phase
   1. Definition
   2. Causes
   3. Management
      a. Therapeutic rest

B. Protracted Active Phase/Primary Dysfunctional Labor
   1. Definition
   2. Causes
   3. Management

C. Secondary Arrest of Dilatation
   1. Definition
   2. Causes
   3. Management

D. Protracted Descent
   1. Definition
   2. Causes
   3. Management

E. Arrest of Descent
   1. Definition
   2. Causes
   3. Management

F. Failure of Descent
   1. Definition
   2. Causes
   3. Management

XIII. Augmentation of Labor

A. Artificial rupture of membranes (AROM)
  1. Indications/Contraindications
  2. Technique
  3. Side effects/potential complications

B. Oxytocin (Pitocin)
  1. Indications/Contraindications
  2. Dose/rate of administration
  3. Side effects/potential complications

XIV. Maternal Exhaustion

A. Signs and symptoms

B. Management

XV. Uterine Rupture

A. Predisposing factors

B. Signs/symptoms/Diagnosis

C. Management

XVI. Shoulder Dystocia

A. Definition

B. Predisposing factors

C. Signs/symptoms/Diagnosis

D. Management

XVII. Compound Presentations

A. Diagnosis

B. Management

XVIII. Abnormal Presentations (Breech, Transverse, Face, Brow)

A. Diagnosis

B. Management

XIX. Multiple Gestation

A. Possible intrapartum complications

B. Monitoring during labor

C. Management

XX. Blood Transfusion Reaction/Anaphylaxis

A. Signs/symptoms/Diagnosis

B. Management

Chapter 13 Questions

Complications of the First and Second Stages of Labor

1. What is the leading cause of perinatal morbidity and mortality in the United States?
   a. Congenital defects
   b. Preterm birth
   c. Infections
   d. Birth trauma/asphyxia

2. A vaginal birth after cesarean section (VBAC) would be MOST likely to be contraindicated for which of the following women?
   a. A woman who had a previous cesarean section for cephalopelvic disproportion (CPD)
   b. A woman with two previous low-transverse cesarean sections for failure to progress
   c. A woman with a previous cesarean section performed using a vertical incision of the lower uterine segment
   d. A woman with a previous emergency cesarean section at 26 weeks before the onset of labor

3. Which of the following statements MOST accurately describes the management of the labor of a woman whom you have determined to be a good candidate for a vaginal birth after cesarean section (VBAC)?
   a. The use of oxytocin for induction or augmentation should be avoided.
   b. The use of epidural anesthesia should be avoided.
   c. She should undergo continuous electronic fetal monitoring.
   d. She should be managed in the same manner as any woman in labor.

DATA FOR ITEM 4

JD is a 27-year-old G2P1 from Brazil. She had a previous cesarean section. From abdominal exam and translations of her medical records that were originally in Portuguese, you have determined it is most likely that she had a classical uterine incision.

4. What is the MOST appropriate management option for JD's delivery?
   a. A scheduled repeat cesarean section without labor
   b. A repeat cesarean section after the onset of labor
   c. A trial of labor for a vaginal delivery
   d. A trial of labor for a vaginal delivery performed in the operating room (OR)

5. Which of the following is the BEST management of an asymptomatic scar dehiscence that occurred during a vaginal birth after cesarean section (VBAC) and that you discover during a postpartum manual exploration of the uterine cavity for retained placental fragments?
   a. Hemabate 250 μg IM
   b. Bimanual compression and uterine massage to avoid hemorrhage
   c. Surgical repair
   d. Nothing, the defect will heal on its own

6. For which of the following women would a diagnosis of preterm labor be accurate?
   a. A woman at 18 weeks gestation with contractions and rupture of membranes
   b. A woman at 24 weeks gestation with contractions every 6 minutes
   c. A woman at 20 weeks gestation with contractions every 8 minutes and rupture of membranes
   d. A woman at 34 weeks gestation with contractions every 10 minutes, 1 centimeter dilation, and

7. Antenatal corticosteroid therapy has been shown to be MOST effective at improving neonatal outcome when administered at what gestational age to women at risk for preterm birth?
   a. 20 to 24 weeks
   b. 24 to 34 weeks
   c. 34 to 36 weeks
   d. 36 to 38 weeks

8. Which of the following is NOT a sequela of preterm birth?
   a. Respiratory distress syndrome
   b. Intraventricular hemorrhage
   c. Low birth weight
   d. Ventricular septal defects

9. Research has demonstrated that which of the following is associated with prevention of preterm labor among women with multiple gestation or a history of preterm labor/birth?
   a. Bed rest especially in a lateral position
   b. Daily contact with a nurse
   c. Prophylactic oral tocolytic therapy
   d. Prophylactic cerclage

10. When performing your initial evaluation of premature rupture of membranes, which of the following should you NOT do?
    a. Sterile speculum examination
    b. Sterile digital vaginal examination
    c. Cervical cultures
    d. Fern test

11. What percentage of women with premature rupture of membranes will go into spontaneous labor within 24 hours?
    a. 45 to 50 percent
    b. 55 to 60 percent
    c. 70 to 75 percent
    d. 80 to 85 percent

12. Which of the following is the MOST technically accurate definition of premature rupture of membranes?
    a. Rupture of membranes before onset of labor
    b. Rupture of membranes more than 24 hours before onset of labor
    c. Rupture of membranes more than 36 hours before onset of labor
    d. Rupture of membranes at less than 36 weeks gestational age

13. Which of the following methods of inducing labor is contraindicated in a woman with premature rupture of membranes?
    a. Castor oil
    b. Nipple stimulation
    c. Sexual intercourse
    d. Oxytocin

14. Which of the following is NOT associated with intrauterine infection?
    a. Fetal tachycardia
    b. Hypertonic uterus
    c. A biophysical profile score of 6 or less (Manning Criteria)
    d. A white blood cell count with a shift to the left

15. In a client with premature rupture of membranes (PROM) at 32 weeks with no current signs of infection, which of the following is the MOST appropriate management plan?

    a. Induction if labor has not initiated spontaneously within 72 hours of PROM because the risk of sepsis outweighs the risks of prematurity

    b. Induction of labor 24 hours after the administration of corticosteroids to promote fetal lung maturity

    c. Watchful waiting and allowing pregnancy to continue for as long as possible because the risks of prematurity outweigh the risks of sepsis

    d. Expectant management at home with cervical cultures and biophysical profiles every 2 weeks

DATA FOR ITEMS 16–17

LK is an 18-year-old G1P0 at 38 weeks gestation. She calls you to report that she has a temperature of 102°F and that she is leaking some liquid that "smells really bad." You have her come into the office and find that in addition to an elevated temperature and foul-smelling vaginal discharge, that her uterus is tender and her heart rate is 100 bpm. Fetal heart rate is 180 bpm.

16. Which of the following is your MOST likely diagnosis?

    a. Pyelonephritis

    b. Salpingitis

    c. Appendicitis

    d. Chorioamnionitis

17. What is the MOST appropriate first step to take at this time?

    a. Admit to the hospital for induced vaginal birth or cesarean section within 24 hours

    b. Admit to the hospital for IV antibiotics and to await onset of labor

    c. Obtain cervical cultures and start empirical oral antibiotic treatment pending culture results

    d. Admit to the hospital for an emergency cesarean section

18. Which is the FIRST step in the management of cord prolapse?

    a. Place the woman in a Trendelenberg or knee-chest position

    b. Give your back-up physician a STAT call

    c. Place your hand into the woman's vagina and hold up the presenting part off the umbilical cord

    d. Wrap the cord loosely with gauze soaked in warm, sterile saline

19. Which of the following is a contraindication for induction of labor?

    a. Chorioamnionitis

    b. Fetal distress

    c. Severe pregnancy induced hypertension

    d. Fetal demise

20. Calculate the Montevideo units for a woman who in the last twenty minutes has had four contractions each 5 minutes apart, lasting 45 seconds, and with a baseline of 10 mmHg and amplitude of 55 mmHg.

    a. 90

    b. 110

    c. 135

    d. 165

21. Why should oxytocin only be administered with a physiologic electrolyte solution such as lactated ringers and not with an aqueous fluid such as dextrose in water?

    a. To avoid uterine hyperstimulation

    b. To avoid incompatibility of the liquids

    c. To avoid water intoxication

    d. To avoid giving a bolus of oxytocin

22. Which of the following contraction patterns defines hyperstimulation of the uterus?
    a. Contractions more frequent than every 3 minutes lasting more than 90 seconds
    b. Contractions more frequent than every 3 minutes lasting more than 60 seconds
    c. Contractions more frequent than every 2 minutes lasting more than 90 seconds
    d. Contractions more frequent than every 2 minutes lasting more than 60 seconds

23. Which of the following statements about fetal tachycardia is FALSE?
    a. Isolated tachycardia is not usually associated with poor fetal outcome.
    b. Tachycardia can be caused by extreme prematurity (28 weeks).
    c. Tachycardia is often caused by the administration of narcotic pain medications.
    d. Tachycardia can be a sign of fetal anemia.

24. Which of the following components of fetal heart rate assessment is the MOST significant indicator of fetal well-being?
    a. Fetal heart rate baseline
    b. Fetal heart rate variability
    c. Fetal heart acceleration patterns
    d. Fetal heart deceleration patterns

25. Research has demonstrated that acceleration of fetal heart rate in response to fetal scalp stimulation is associated with which of the following?
    a. An immature fetal autonomous nervous system
    b. A fetal blood pH of greater than 7.25
    c. Fetal hypoxia
    d. An intact neurological system

26. What is the most common cause of fetal heart rate acceleration pattern?
    a. Maternal intake of liquids
    b. Hypoxia
    c. Fetal movement
    d. Head compression

27. Which of the following periodic fetal heart changes does not reflect the shape of the uterine contractions?
    a. Early decelerations
    b. Late decelerations
    c. Variable decelerations

28. During which of the following deceleration patterns is the fetal heart rate MOST likely to dip below 100 bpm?
    a. Early deceleration
    b. Late deceleration
    c. Variable deceleration

29. Which of the following is a TRUE statement about late decelerations?
    a. A deeper deceleration is more serious than a shallow deceleration.
    b. They usually start after the acme of the contraction and last more than 90 seconds.
    c. They may occur within the normal heart rate range and be as shallow as 10 bpm.
    d. They usually start once the contraction has ended.

30. Variable decelerations are thought to be caused by which of the following?
    a. Impending birth
    b. Head compression
    c. Uteroplacental insufficiency
    d. Cord compression

31. Late decelerations are thought to be caused by which of the following?
- **a.** Impending birth
- **b.** Head compression
- **c.** Uteroplacental insufficiency
- **d.** Cord compression

DATA FOR ITEMS 32–33

The electronic fetal monitoring strip for a woman in transition reveals repeated variable decelerations down to 60 to 70 bpm with brisk return to a baseline of 140 bpm. There are no other deceleration patterns and there is good variability of the fetal heart rate. Your vaginal exam reveals that the station is +1. There is no evidence of a prolapsed cord.

32. Which of the following interventions is MOST appropriate at this time?
- **a.** Call the physician and prepare for a probable instrument delivery
- **b.** Perform an amniotomy to expedite delivery
- **c.** Change the mother's position
- **d.** Administer oxygen to the mother with a well-fitting face mask at 6–8 L/min

33. Which of the following complications would be MOST likely to be associated with the above fetal heart rate pattern?
- **a.** Nuchal cord
- **b.** Fetal anemia
- **c.** Postmaturity
- **d.** Prematurity

34. In the absence of administration of any medications, a sinusoidal pattern of the fetal heart rate is associated with which of the following?
- **a.** Cord compression
- **b.** Head compression
- **c.** Descent of the fetal head
- **d.** Severe fetal hypoxia

35. What is the definition of hypoxia?
- **a.** Decreased oxygen in the blood
- **b.** Decreased oxygen in the tissue
- **c.** Excessive acidity of the blood
- **d.** Decreased oxygen in the tissue and metabolic acidosis

36. What is the definition of asphyxia?
- **a.** Decreased oxygen in the blood
- **b.** Decreased oxygen in the tissue
- **c.** Excessive acidity of the blood
- **d.** Decreased oxygen in the tissue and metabolic acidosis

37. Which of the following statements about cephalopelvic disproportion (CPD) is TRUE?
- **a.** If the possibility of CPD is strongly suspected, labor is contraindicated.
- **b.** A cesarean delivery is indicated for a woman who had CPD with a previous pregnancy.
- **c.** CPD is a relative determination based on fetal and maternal pelvic size.
- **d.** The only effective therapeutic measures once CPD is diagnosed are operative delivery or cesarean section.

38. Deep transverse arrest is associated with which of the following?
- **a.** Platypelloid pelvic type
- **b.** Uterine hypertonic contractions
- **c.** Breech presentation
- **d.** Synclitism

■   DATA FOR ITEMS 39–40

Upon vaginal examination of a woman in second stage of labor with hypotonic uterine dysfunction, you determine that the saggital suture is in the transverse diameter of the mother's pelvis and that there is considerable molding and formation of caput succedaneum.

39. Which of the following is your MOST likely diagnosis?
    a. Posterior asynclitism
    b. Transverse lie
    c. Fetal malpresentation
    d. Deep transverse arrest

40. Which of the following is NOT part of the management plan for the above situation?
    a. Conduction anesthesia
    b. Change in maternal position
    c. Pitocin
    d. Instrument or cesarean delivery if condition is not overcome

41. What is the usual management for hypertonic uterine dysfunction in early labor?
    a. Administration of morphine and/or a barbiturate
    b. Subcutaneous or IV terbutaline
    c. Pitocin
    d. Cesarean section

■   DATA FOR ITEM 42

A multipara in first stage of labor has had no change in cervical dilation in 3 hours. You have ensured maternal hydration, encouraged ambulation, and performed an amniotomy which revealed clear amniotic fluid.

42. If the above measures do not achieve progressive cervical dilation, what is the MOST appropriate step to take next?
    a. Prepare the woman for an instrument delivery
    b. Prepare the woman for a cesarean section
    c. Continue with watchful waiting
    d. Pitocin stimulation

■   DATA FOR ITEMS FOR 43–44

A woman in labor experiences a sharp pain at the peak of one of her contractions after which her contractions stop and she begins bleeding vaginally. There are sudden, severe and repeated fetal heart decelerations and there is a fetal loss of station.

43. What is the MOST likely diagnosis in this case?
    a. Amniotic fluid embolism
    b. Placental abruption
    c. Uterine rupture
    d. Vasa previa

44. In addition to alerting the physician STAT, what is the MOST important action for the midwife to take NEXT in this situation?
    a. Prepare the woman for immediate delivery
    b. Order blood for a transfusion and ensure that there is appropriate venous access
    c. Institute aortic compression and add an oxytotic to the IV solution
    d. Prepare for a full-scale neonatal resuscitation effort

45. Which of the following is diagnostic of shoulder dystocia?
   a. Extreme difficulty with the delivery of the fetal shoulders
   b. Wedging of the anterior shoulder above the symphysis pubis
   c. Wedging of the posterior shoulder above the sacral promontory
   d. Wedging of the posterior shoulder against the sacrum

46. The fetal shoulders normally enter the true pelvis with the bisacromial diameter in which of the following diameters?
   a. Transverse
   b. Oblique
   c. Anteroposterior

47. Which of the following defines Varney's predictive factor for shoulder dystocia?
   a. The presence of an indication for the need for a midpelvic rotation or delivery
   b. A pelvic shape that significantly decreases the anterior-posterior diameter of the pelvis
   c. An estimated fetal weight 1 pound or more greater than the woman's largest previous baby
   d. A desultory active phase of labor combined with a prolonged second stage of labor

48. It is believed that the exaggerated lithotomy position (McRoberts maneuver) facilitates delivery of the fetal shoulders through which of the following mechanisms?
   a. Increasing the length of the anteroposterior pelvic diameter
   b. Producing rotation of the shoulders into an oblique diameter
   c. Increasing the room for the attendant to deliver the shoulders
   d. Rotating the symphysis pubis to free the impacted shoulder

49. Which of the following is NOT an appropriate procedure to manage a shoulder dystocia?
   a. Manual rotation of the shoulders
   b. Supra-pubic pressure
   c. Fundal pressure
   d. Episiotomy

50. Birth in a face presentation is only possible if internal rotation brings the mentum (chin) into which of the following positions?
   a. Anterior
   b. Posterior
   c. Transverse
   d. Oblique

51. During a breech delivery, a hands-off approach is recommended until the baby is born spontaneously up to which body part?
   a. The sacrum
   b. The umbilicus
   c. The scapula
   d. The nape of the neck

52. During a breech delivery, suprapubic pressure is applied for which of the following reasons?
   a. To avoid an impacting of the shoulders
   b. To facilitate delivery of the sacrum
   c. To avoid impacting of the bitrochanteric fetal diameter
   d. To maintain flexion of the fetal head

53. What is the reasoning behind immediately clamping and cutting the cord of the first-born twin?
   a. To avoid cord entanglement/compression by the second fetus
   b. To avoid having the second twin exsanguinate through the cord
   c. To avoid having the first twin exsanguinate through the cord
   d. To avoid premature separation of the placenta

54. Which of the following findings does NOT on its own signal fetal hypoxemia?
   a. Persistent late decelerations
   b. Meconium-stained amniotic fluid
   c. Sustained loss of variability
   d. Wandering baseline

55. Which of the following is NOT a contraindication for tocolysis?
   a. Fetal maturity
   b. Acute fetal distress
   c. Chorioamnionitis
   d. Gestational diabetes mellitus

Chapter 13 Answer Key

Complications of the First and Second Stages of Labor

1. *b* p. 461

2. *d* p. 459–460

3. *d* p. 461

4. *a* p. 460

5. *d* p. 461

6. *c* p. 463

7. *b* p. 465

8. *d* p. 465

9. *b* p. 463

10. *b* p. 467

11. *d* p. 468

12. *a* p. 467

13. *c* p. 469

14. *b* p. 469

15. *c* p. 470

16. *d* p. 470–471

17. *a* p. 471

18. *c* p. 472

19. *b* p. 473

20. *a* p. 475

21. *c* p. 475

22. *c* p. 475

23. *c* p. 476

24. *b* p. 476–477

25. *b* p. 477

26. *c* p. 477

27. *c* p. 478–479

28. *c* p. 479–480

29. *c* p. 478

30. *d* p. 479

31. *c* p. 478

32. *c* p. 480

33. *a* p. 479

34. *d* p. 481

35. *b* p. 482

36. *d* p. 482

37. *c* p. 483

38. *a* p. 485

39. *d* p. 485

40. *a* p. 485

41. *a* p. 487

42. *d* p. 487

43. *c* p. 488

44. *b* p. 488

45. *b* p. 493

46. *b* p. 493

47. *c* p. 495

48. *d* p. 496

49. *c* p. 496

50. *a* p. 501

51. *b* p. 504

52. *d* p. 507

53. *b* p. 510

54. *b* p. 483

55. *d* p. 464

Chapter 14 Outline
The Normal Third and Fourth Stages of Labor

I.   Third Stage of Labor

  A. Definition

  B. Parameters of normal/Friedman Curve

II.   Maternal and Newborn Assessment During the Third Stage of Labor

III. Delivery of Placenta

  A. Signs of Placental Separation

  B. Technique
   1. Guarding the uterus
   2. Modified Brandt-Andrews maneuver
   3. Brandt-Andrews maneuver
   4. Controlled-cord traction

  C. Shultz vs. Duncan mechanisms

  D. Trailing membranes

  E. Use of oxytotics

IV.   Fourth Stage of Labor

  A. Definition

  B. Parameters of normal

V.   Assessment of Maternal and Neonatal Status in the Fourth Stage

VI.   Assessment of Maternal and Neonatal Bonding

VII. Assessment of the Uterus

  A. Uterine tone

  B. Fundal height

VIII. Assessment of Vagina and Perineum

  A. Definition:
   1. First degree lacerations
   2. Second degree lacerations
   3. Third degree lacerations
   4. Fourth degree lacerations
   5. Sulcus tears
   6. Periurethral lacerations

IX.   Assessment/Inspection of the Cervix and Upper Vaginal Vault

    A. Indications

    B. Technique

X.   Repair of Episiotomy or Lacerations

    A. Relevant anatomy (pelvic muscles and structures)

    B. Indications

    C. Technique (including choice of suture material, needle, gauge, and type of stitches)

XI.   Inspection of the Placenta, Membranes, and Cord

    A. Technique

    B. Parameters of normal/Variations of Normal

    C. Significance of placental/cord abnormalities

Chapter 14 Questions
Normal Third and Fourth Stages of Labor

1. What is the average duration of the third stage of labor?
   a. 1 to 5 minutes
   b. 5 to 10 minutes
   c. 10 to 15 minutes
   d. 15 to 20 minutes

2. In addition to uterine contractions, which of the following mechanisms is responsible for placental separation?
   a. The abrupt decrease in the size of the uterine cavity
   b. Tension placed on the cord by the birth of the baby
   c. Bleeding into the intervillous space which releases prostaglandins
   d. The constriction of blood vessels that provided circulation to the placenta

3. Once you are sure that the placenta has separated, what is the next step you should take in managing the delivery of the placenta?
   a. Apply controlled cord traction
   b. Assess whether the uterus is contracted
   c. Apply fundal pressure to propel the placenta through the vaginal canal
   d. Administer an IM or IV oxytocic agent

4. After the placenta separates and moves into the lower uterine segment or the upper vaginal vault, which of the following changes in the uterus would you expect?
   a. It would fall in the abdomen as the process of involution begins
   b. It would be displaced upward and thus rise in the abdomen
   c. It would be displaced sideways and thus be felt in the right or left quadrants
   d. It would remain midline in the abdomen and at the same height but become firmer

■ DATA FOR ITEM 5

As the placenta is expelled you notice that the maternal side of the placenta is presenting.

5. Which of the following statements is true about this type of placental presentation?
   a. It is called the Schultz mechanism and results from placental separation that begins centrally.
   b. It is called the Duncan mechanism and results from placental separation that begins centrally.
   c. It is called the Schultz mechanism and results from separation that begins at the margin or periphery of the placenta.
   d. It is called the Duncan mechanism and results from a separation that begins at the margin or periphery of the placenta.

6. Which of the following describes the modified Brandt-Andrews maneuver?
   a. Bringing the fingertips of your abdominal hand straight down above the symphysis into the lower abdomen while holding the umbilical cord taut to check for placental separation
   b. Pushing down and toward the umbilicus on the uterus above the symphysis pubis with the palm of your abdominal hand to facilitate placental expulsion after separation
   c. Keeping a hand on the uterine fundus to ascertain shape, position, and consistency of the uterus and prevent premature fundal massage
   d. Exerting pressure on the fundus after placental expulsion to ensure that any clots that may interfere with proper uterine involution are expelled

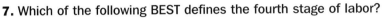
7. Which of the following BEST defines the fourth stage of labor?

    a. The period beginning with the birth of the placenta and ending when the uterus remains well-contracted and vaginal bleeding is minimal

    b. The period beginning with the birth of the placenta and ending one hour later

    c. The period beginning with the birth of the placenta and ending 24 hours later

    d. The period beginning with the birth of the placenta and ending when both the mother and the fetus are in stable condition

8. A woman's blood pressure, pulse, and respirations should be monitored how often during the normal fourth stage of labor?

    a. At least every 15 minutes until stable at prelabor levels

    b. At least every 30 minutes until stable at prelabor levels

    c. Immediately after the birth of the placenta and then again every 30 minutes for 4 hours

    d. At least every hour for 24 hours

■ DATA FOR ITEM 9

You are creating a management plan for the fourth stage of labor for a woman who just delivered a term 4200 g infant following a prolonged first stage of labor for which you initiated Pitocin. The second stage of labor was unremarkable except for the fact that you performed an episiotomy to expedite the birth of the infant's head.

9. You know that this woman is at MOST risk for which of the following complications of the fourth stage of labor?

    a. Retained placental fragments

    b. Uterine relaxation/atony

    c. Hemorrhage from a cervical laceration

    d. Hematoma

10. All of the following would be indications for postpartum inspection of the cervix EXCEPT:

    a. Following a twin or breech birth

    b. A well contracted uterus accompanied by a steady trickle of blood from the vagina

    c. The presence of an anterior lip that had to be pushed back manually

    d. A forceps or vacuum extraction delivery

Chapter 14 Answer Key
The Third and Fourth Stages of Labor

1. *b* p. 513

2. *a* p. 513

3. *b* p. 517

4. *b* p. 513

5. *d* p. 514

6. *a* p. 516

7. *b* p. 525

8. *a* p. 528

9. *b* p. 526–527

10. *a* p. 527

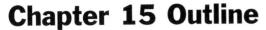

Chapter 15 Outline
Complications of the Third and Fourth Stages of Labor

I. Retained Placenta

    A. Definition

    B. Predisposing factors/Causes

    C. Management
        1. Manual removal of the placenta

II. Third Stage Hemorrhage

    A. Definition

    B. Predisposing factors/Causes

    C. Management
        1. Manual removal of the placenta/Manual uterine exploration
        2. Use of oxytotics

III. Placenta Accreta

    A. Definition

    B. Predisposing factors

    C. Diagnosis

    D. Management

IV. Uterine Inversion

    A. Definition

    B. Predisposing factors/Causes

    C. Management
        1. Manual reposition of the uterus

V. Immediate Postpartum Hemorrhage

    A. Definition

    B. Predisposing factors/Causes

    C. Management
        1. Use of oxytocics
            a. Indications/Contraindications
            b. Type, dose, route, side effects, potential complications
        2. Bimanual compression

Chapter 15 Questions
Complications of the Third and Fourth Stages of Labor

■   **DATA FOR ITEM 1**

As you try to tease out trailing membranes during third stage, you feel that there is some tearing of the membranes. You inspect the placenta and the membranes and it appears that parts of the membranes are indeed missing and, therefore, probably retained within the uterus.

1. What is the MOST appropriate management of this situation?
   a. Perform a manual uterine examination and removal of retained membranes to ensure that a hemorrhage does not ensue
   b. Order a course of prophylactic penicillin to avoid infection due to retained membrane fragments
   c. Order a Methergine series for the woman to achieve rapid expulsion of retained membrane fragments
   d. Contact consulting physician for uterine exploration and possible surgical removal of retained membranes

2. What is the MOST common cause of third stage hemorrhage?
   a. Mismanagement of third stage
   b. Uterine atony
   c. Cervical lacerations
   d. Retained placental fragments

■   **DATA FOR ITEMS 3–4**

As you examine a placenta during the postpartum period you notice approximately four, small, hard, nodular, whitish areas on both the maternal and fetal side of the placenta.

3. What is the term used to describe these nodules?
   a. Infarcts
   b. Calcifications
   c. Inclusion cysts
   d. Succenturiate lobes

4. What is the MOST appropriate management of this finding?
   a. Note it as a normal degenerative change of the placenta
   b. Send the placenta to pathology for detailed examination
   c. Obtain a culture from the area around the nodes to screen for infection
   d. Notify the pediatrician because these nodules are associated with kidney abnormalities in the newborn

5. What is the MAIN clinical significance of lobulated and succenturiate placentas?
   a. That they are associated with an increase in fetal anomalies
   b. That they are often seen in women with severe preeclampsia or eclampsia
   c. That placental lobes may be retained and not expelled with the rest of the placenta
   d. That it is a sign of uterine pathology

■ **DATA FOR ITEM 6**

As you examine a placenta following a normal birth, you note that the umbilical cord inserts in the edge, or margin, of the placenta.

6. This is referred to as which of the following?
   a. Battledore placenta
   b. Velamentous insertion
   c. Placenta marginata
   d. Vasa previa

7. Approximately what percentage of infants born with only one umbilical artery will have multiple, severe malformations?
   a. 10%
   b. 20%
   c. 30%
   d. 40%

■ **DATA FOR ITEMS 8–9**

You are called in to assist in management of a third stage hemorrhage due to partial placental separation. You immediately put a STAT call in to the consulting physician, and as you come into the room, you notice that there is an IV line running with Ringer's lactate.

8. What is the BEST action to take at this point to manage the hemorrhage?
   a. Massage the uterus to attempt to complete the placental separation and then apply controlled cord traction to facilitate delivery of the placenta
   b. Ensure an empty bladder to provide some IV analgesia and manually remove the placenta
   c. Apply bi-manual uterine compression to stop the hemorrhage
   d. Add some oxytocin to the IV infusion to promote uterine contraction to cause placental separation

9. The partial placental separation that led to this third stage hemorrhage was MOST likely due to which of the following?
   a. Uterine massage prior to placental separation
   b. Partial placenta accreta
   c. Retroplacental hematoma
   d. Premature and excessive cord traction

10. What is the MOST appropriate management of placenta accreta?
   a. Attempt a manual removal of the placenta
   b. Apply controlled cord traction while supporting to uterine fundus to avoid uterine inversion
   c. Administer either methergine or hemabate
   d. Contact the physician and prepare the woman for immediate surgery

11. Which of the following statements regarding manual repositioning of the uterus following uterine inversion is TRUE?
   a. It can only be performed by a physician.
   b. It requires the administration of medication such as terbutaline to stop uterine contractions.
   c. It can be performed regardless of the time lapse between inversion and diagnosis.
   d. It should be performed with the placenta still attached to the uterine wall.

12. What is the LAST step in manual removal of placenta?
   a. Examination of the placenta to see that it is complete and intact
   b. Uterine exploration to ensure that there has been complete removal of the placenta
   c. Thorough fundal/uterine massage to ensure that the uterus is contracted
   d. Administration of oxytocin

13. What is the MOST common cause of immediate postpartum hemorrhage?
    a. Mismanagement of the third stage of labor
    b. Uterine atony
    c. Cervical or vaginal lacerations
    d. Oxytocin induction or augmentation

14. What is the proper dosage and frequency for a methylergonovine (Methergine) series?
    a. 0.2 mg every 4 hours for 6 doses
    b. 0.2 mg every 6 hours for 4 doses
    c. 0.4 mg every 4 hours for 6 doses
    d. 0.4 mg every 6 hours for 4 doses

■ DATA FOR ITEM 15

As you examine a placenta, you note that there appear to be several cotyledons missing.

15. What is the MOST appropriate management of this situation?
    a. Perform a manual uterine examination and removal of the retained placental fragments to ensure that a hemorrhage does not ensue.
    b. Order a course of prophylactic penicillin to avoid infection due to the retained placental fragments.
    c. Order IM Methergine to achieve rapid expulsion of the retained placental fragments.
    d. Contact consulting physician for uterine exploration and possible surgical removal of the retained placental fragments.

16. Which of the following is the widely accepted definition of postpartum hemorrhage?
    a. Loss of 400 mL of blood or greater
    b. Loss of 500 mL of blood or greater
    c. Loss of 800 mL of blood or greater
    d. Loss of 1000 mL of blood or greater

17. What is the drug of choice for a normotensive woman who is experiencing excessive postpartum bleeding due to uterine atony?
    a. A synthetic oxytocin (Pitocin, Oxytocin, Syntocinon)
    b. Methylergonovine maleate (Methergine)
    c. Prostaglandin F2 alpha (Hemabate)
    d. Prostaglandin E2 (Dinoprostone)

■ DATA FOR ITEM 18

When you perform a uterine check on a woman that is in the immediate postpartum stage, you note that her uterus is atonic and that she has a steady flow of blood from the vagina. You begin uterine massage, but despite the massage the uterus fails to contract.

18. Other than ordering some IM Pitocin, what is the MOST appropriate action to take next?
    a. Continue with the uterine massage while you wait for the Pitocin to take effect
    b. Begin bimanual uterine compression
    c. Perform a uterine exploration for placental fragments or cotyledons
    d. Quickly but thoroughly examine the woman for cervical, vaginal, and perineal lacerations

19. Which of the following pelvic muscles comprises the largest portion of the pelvic floor?
    a. Deep transverse perineal
    b. Superficial transverse perineal
    c. Pubococcygeus
    d. Levator ani

20. Which of the following muscles would NOT be cut in a midline episiotomy?

   a. Bulbocavernosus
   b. Pubococcygeus
   c. Superficial transverse perineal
   d. Deep transverse perineal

21. Which of the following statements is TRUE regarding mediolateral episiotomies?

   a. Since they are longer cuts, they are more likely to extend into the rectal sphincter and the rectum.
   b. They are less painful than a midline episiotomy because there are fewer nerve branches in the area that is cut and repaired.
   c. They are easier to repair than a midline episiotomy because there is a decreased risk of entering the rectum during the repair.
   d. They are indicated if there is an increased risk of a severe laceration or cut that will extend into the rectal sphincter and rectum.

DATA FOR ITEM 22

As you examine a woman's vagina and perineum during the fourth stage of labor, you notice that she has a laceration that involves the vaginal mucosa, posterior fourchette, perineal skin, and perineal muscles.

22. This laceration is classified as which of the following?

   a. A first degree laceration
   b. A second degree laceration
   c. A third degree laceration
   d. A fourth degree laceration

23. What gauge suture should you use to repair a tear/incision of the vaginal mucosa?

   a. 2–0
   b. 3–0
   c. 4–0
   d. 5–0

24. What gauge suture should you use to repair a clitoral tear?

   a. 2–0
   b. 3–0
   c. 4–0
   d. 5–0

25. A sulcus tear is which of the following type of laceration?

   a. First degree laceration
   b. Second degree laceration
   c. Third degree laceration
   d. Fourth degree laceration

Chapter 15 Answer Key

Complications of the Third and Fourth Stages of Labor

1. *c* p. 518

2. *a* p. 515, 521

3. *a* p. 835

4. *a* p. 835

5. *c* p. 836

6. *a* p. 837

7. *c* p. 837

8. *a* p. 522

9. *a* p. 521

10. *d* p. 522

11. *d* p. 523

12. *d* p. 844

13. *b* p. 525, 531

14. *a* p. 518

15. *a* p. 534

16. *b* p. 531

17. *b* p. 532

18. *b* p. 533

19. *d* p. 849

20. *b* p. 853

21. *d* p. 447

22. *b* p. 864

23. *b* p. 860

24. *c* p. 859, 866

25. *b* p. 864

PART V: CARE OF THE NEWBORN

PART V

Chapter 16 Outline
Transition of the Fetus to Extrauterine Life

I. Respiratory Changes

    A. Physiology of the first breath/Maintenance of respirations

    B. Normal respiratory responses/characteristics of the newborn

    C. Signs/symptoms of abnormal respiratory transition

II. Circulatory Changes

    A. Fetal circulation

    B. Transition from fetal to neonatal circulation

    C. Signs/symptoms of abnormal circulatory transition

III. Thermoregulation

    A. Brown fat/Non-shivering thermogenesis

    B. Methods of heat loss (convection, radiation, evaporation, conduction)

    C. Methods to minimize heat loss in the newborn

    D. Hypothermia
        1. Signs/symptoms
        2. Management
        3. Possible sequelae
        4. Interaction/relation to hypoglycemia and respiratory distress

IV. Glucose Regulation

    A. Normal glucose regulation in the newborn

    B. Methods to promote euglycemia in the newborn

    C. Hypoglycemia
        1. Signs/symptoms
        2. Management
            a. Obtaining a blood glucose level
        3. Possible sequelae
        4. Interaction/relation to hypothermia and respiratory distress

V. Changes in Blood

    A. Normal blood lab values of a full-term infant

VI.   Changes in Gastrointestinal System

A. Adaptations to exogenous food sources

B. Passage of meconium

C. Gut closure

VII.   Changes in the Immune System

A. Natural vs. Acquired immunity

B. Active vs. Passive immunity

VIII.   Changes in the Renal System

Chapter 16 Questions
Transition of the Fetus to Extrauterine Life

1. Which of the following has the potential to inhibit respirations in the newborn?
   a. Rubbing on the newborn's back
   b. Flicking the sole of the newborn's foot
   c. Exposure of the newborn to cold
   d. Exposure of the newborn to light and noise

2. What is the function of surfactant in the lungs of the newborn?
   a. Reducing the pressure needed for respiration by stabilizing the walls of the alveoli
   b. Promoting decreased pulmonary vascular resistance and increased pulmonary perfusion
   c. Causing an increase in the systemic vascular resistance
   d. Pushing fluid within the lungs to the periphery where it is absorbed, allowing the alveoli to expand

3. Which of the following is an abnormal respiratory response of the newborn as it transitions to extrauterine life?
   a. A respiratory rate of 58 breaths per minute with diaphragmatic breathing
   b. Obligate nose breathing that sounds noisy and wet
   c. A respiratory rate of 56 breaths per minute with abdominal breathing
   d. Retractions of the intercostal muscles

4. What is the effect on the newborn's cardiovascular system of clamping of the umbilical cord?
   a. Decreasing systemic vascular resistance
   b. Increasing systemic vascular resistance
   c. Increasing pulmonary vascular resistance
   d. Decreasing pulmonary vascular resistance

5. Which of the following neonatal heat-creating mechanisms is MOST efficient?
   a. Muscle flexion
   b. Shivering
   c. Non-shivering thermogenesis
   d. Voluntary muscle activity

■ DATA FOR ITEM 6

You are trying to re-warm a newborn who has been stressed by hypothermia by placing her under a radiant warmer.

6. Which of the following actions will be MOST helpful in safely and effectively accomplishing the re-warming process?
   a. Uncover the newborn's head prior to placing her under the warmer
   b. Keep the infant's head covered while she is under the warmer
   c. Keep the newborn's body wrapped while she is under the warmer
   d. Adjust the temperature on the warmer so that the re-warming process occurs within 15–30 minutes

7. What is the mean glucose level for newborns from 4 to 72 hours after birth?
   a. 50–60 mg/dL
   b. 60–70 mg/dL
   c. 70–80 mg/dL
   d. 80–90 mg/dL

8. Which of the following BEST describes the process of gluconeongenesis?
   a. The production of glucose through the utilization of breastmilk/formula
   b. Production of glucose through anaerobic metabolism
   c. Production of glucose through the use of glycogen stores
   d. Production of glucose from body sources other than glycogen

9. The short life span of the newborn's red blood cells leads to quick cell turnover which, in turn, leads to which of the following?
   a. A low reticulocyte count
   b. Transient newborn anemia
   c. Physiologic jaundice
   d. Peripheral cyanosis

10. What is the approximate maximum capacity of the stomach of the term newborn?
   a. 20 cc
   b. 30 cc
   c. 50 cc
   d. 60 cc

11. Which of the following characteristics of the newborn gastrointestinal system predisposes the newborn to water loss complications?
   a. The impaired ability of the newborn to digest proteins and fats
   b. The incomplete juncture of the lower esophagus and the stomach
   c. The immaturity of the intestinal epithelium
   d. The immaturity of the lining of the colon

12. Which of the following BEST describes the process of "gut closure"?
   a. Process by which the epithelial surfaces of the intestine become impermeable to antigens
   b. Process by which the surfaces of the large intestine gain the capability to produce certain clotting factors
   c. Process by which the epithelial cells of the intestine mature and gain the ability for effective absorption of nutrients
   d. Process by which the epithelial cells of the intestine gain the capability to produce substances such as trypsin and amalyse, which assist in digestion

◼ **DATA FOR ITEM 13**

The umbilical cord blood of a newborn born to a mother who was exposed to CMV infection during pregnancy is sent to the lab for analysis.

13. Which of the following findings would suggest that the fetus has actively responded to a CMV infection in utero?
   a. Postitive IgG antibodies to CMV
   b. Positive IgM antibodies to CMV
   c. The presence of polymorphonuclear neutrophils (PMN's)
   d. The presence of macrophages

14. Metabolic acidosis caused by cold stress has which of the following effects on the pulmonary vasculature?
   a. Left to right shunting
   b. Right to left shunting
   c. Vasoconstriction
   d. Vasodilation

15. The fetal lungs require all of the following for the production of surfactant EXCEPT:
    a. Oxygen
    b. Glucose
    c. Lactic acid
    d. Lung perfusion

16. Which of the following statements about brown adipose tissue (BAT) is TRUE?
    a. There is more of it present in infants with postmaturity syndrome
    b. It is a renewable source of heat production for the newborn
    c. It is located throughout the subcutaneous layer of the skin in the newborn
    d. Its utilization is under the control of the hypothalamus and is triggered by cold stimulus.

17. Which of the following is MOST directly responsible for closure of the foramen ovale?
    a. Decrease in blood pH
    b. Increase in lymph circulation
    c. Increased pressure in the left atrium
    d. Increase in oxygen levels in the blood

Chapter 16 Answer Key

Transition of the Fetus to Extrauterine Life

1. *c* p. 552

2. *a* p. 552

3. *d* p. 552

4. *b* p. 553

5. *c* p. 554

6. *a* p. 555

7. *b* p. 555

8. *d* p. 555

9. *c* p. 557

10. *b* p. 557

11. *d* p. 558

12. *a* p. 558

13. *b* p. 558

14. *c* p. 554

15. *c* p. 554

16. *d* p. 554

17. *c* p. 553

Chapter 17 Outline
The Healthy Newborn

I. **Apgar Scores**

II. **Transitional Period**

    A. First period of reactivity

    B. Period of unresponsive sleep

    C. Second period of reactivity

        1. Timing/duration of each period

        2. Characteristics of each period

            a. Motor activity/muscle tone

            b. Color

            c. Respirations

            d. Heart sounds

            e. Mucus

            f. Bowel

III. **Vital Sign Assessment/Signs and Symptoms of Normal Transition**

    A. Tone

    B. Reflexes

    C. Behavior

    D. Bowel sounds

    E. Pulse

    F. Respirations/Breath sounds

    G. Temperature

    H. Glucose levels

    I. Hematocrit levels

IV. **Thermoregulation (Discussed further in Chapters 16 and 18)**

V. **Eye Prophylaxis**

VI. **Vitamin K Administration**

VII. **Feedings**

    A. Timing

    B. Duration

    C. Frequency

VIII. Urination and Stools

    A. Meconium

    B. Frequency

    C. Character

IX. Skin Care

X. Promoting Infant-Maternal/Family Bonding

    A. The first feed

    B. Rooming-in

XI. Preparations for Discharge from Hospital/Birth-Center

Chapter 17 Questions
The Healthy Newborn

1. Which of the following statements about the Apgar scoring system is TRUE?
   a. It was developed as a predictor of neurological damage.
   b. It can be used to determine the need for and success of resuscitation efforts.
   c. It is used at birth, 1 minute, and five minutes of life.
   d. It evaluates the same basic criteria as the biophysical profile.

DATA FOR ITEM 2

A newborn under your care exhibits the following at 1 minute following birth:

Heart rate of 88 bpm

Slow, irregular breathing with grunting

Limp extremities

A grimace in response to stimulus

Pale color

2. What is this newborn's Apgar score?
   a. 3
   b. 4
   c. 5
   d. 6

DATA FOR ITEM 3

A newborn under your care exhibits the following at 1 minute after birth:

Heart rate of 116

Vigorous, wet-sounding crying

Active motion of extremities

Pink body, blue feet and hands

3. What is this newborn's Apgar score?
   a. 7
   b. 8
   c. 9
   d. 10

4. Which of the following findings would be considered ABNORMAL in a newborn at 10 minutes following birth?
   a. Heart rate of 178 when crying
   b. Acrocyanosis
   c. Rales and rhonchi of the lungs
   d. Decreased muscle tone and jitteriness

5. Which of the following findings would be considered ABNORMAL in a newborn at 4 hours following birth?
   a. Variable heart rate and swift changes in color
   b. Rales or rhonchi of the lungs
   c. Variable respiratory rate
   d. Spitting up of milk and mucus after feedings

6. What is the maximum amount of time after birth that a newborn can go without voiding before referral to a pediatric provider is warranted?

   a. 12 hours
   b. 24 hours
   c. 48 hours
   d. 72 hours

7. Which of the following BEST describes the reasoning behind administering Vitamin K to newborns?

   a. Because the newborn liver, where clotting factors are manufactured, is immature
   b. Because the trauma of birth quickly exhausts the available clotting factors in the newborn's reserve
   c. Because the newborn gut, where Vitamin K is synthesized, is immature
   d. Because Vitamin K protects against bacterial colonization of the newborn's gut

8. Which of the following offers the best protection against opthalmic infections caused by gonorrhea or chlamydia?

   a. 0.5% Silver nitrate drops
   b. 1% Silver nitrate drops
   c. 0.5% Erythromycin ointment
   d. 1% Erythromycin ointment

9. Which of the following would be the BEST time to apply eye prophylaxis against opthalmic infection by gonorrhea or chlamydia?

   a. Immediately after birth
   b. Within the first 30 minutes following birth
   c. At approximately 1 to 2 hours following birth
   d. 24 hours after birth

10. Which of the following would be the BEST time for a healthy newborn to attempt breast-feeding for the first time?

   a. Within the first 30 minutes of life
   b. Sometime between 30 minutes and 2 hours of age
   c. During the second period of reactivity
   d. Sometime between 2 and 6 hours of age

Chapter 17 Answer Key
The Healthy Newborn

   1. *b* p. 562

   2. *a* p. 562

   3. *c* p. 562

   4. *d* p. 563

   5. *b* p. 564

   6. *b* p. 565

   7. *c* p. 565

   8. *c* p. 565

   9. *c* p. 565

   10. *a* p. 563

Chapter 18 Outline
Neonatal Resuscitation

I.   Pre-delivery preparations

   A. Equipment and Supplies

   B. Anticipating asphyxia/need for resuscitation
      1. Common causes of respiratory depression at birth

   C. Delegation/Delineation of responsibilities

II.   Asphyxia

   A. Pathophysiology

   B. Signs/Symptoms of asphyxia
      1. Primary vs. secondary apnea

   C. Effects of hypoxia

III.   Process of Resuscitation

   A. ABC's of Resuscitation
      1. Airway
      2. Breathing
      3. Circulation

   B. Thermoregulation/Warming of the Newborn

   C. Opening the Airway
      1. Positioning
      2. Bulb syringe suctioning
         a. Indications
         b. Technique
      3. Suctioning with suction catheter
         a. Indications
         b. Technique
      4. Suctioning of the trachea
         a. Indications
         b. Technique

   D. Evaluation of the Infant
      1. Respirations
      2. Heart rate
      3. Color

   E. Tactile stimulation of the newborn
      1. Indications
      2. Technique

   F. Free-Flow Oxygen
      1. Indications

2. Technique

    a. Mask vs. Tubing

G. Positive Pressure Ventilation

    1. Indications

    2. Technique

        a. Anesthesia bag vs. self-inflating bag

        b. Resuscitation masks

        c. Ventilation rate/ventilation pressures

        d. Reevaluation of respirations/heart rate

H. Chest Compressions

    1. Indications

    2. Technique

        a. Positioning

        b. Compression rate

        c. Ventilation during chest compressions

        d. Reevaluation of heart rate/respirations

I. Endotracheal Intubation

    1. Indications

    2. Technique

        a. Supplies

        b. Anatomy

        c. Positioning

        d. Inserting the laryngoscope

        e. Placing the ET tube

        f. Confirming ET tube placement

J. Medications

    1. Epinephrine

    2. Volume expanders

    3. Sodium bicarbonate

    4. Naloxone hydrochloride

    Know the following for all of the above medications:

        a. Indications

        b. Concentration

        c. Preparation

        d. Dosage/Route

        e. Rate/Precautions

K.   **Orogastric Catheter**

    1. Indications

    2. Technique

IV. **Care of the Neonate Born in Meconium-Stained Fluid**

A. Suctioning

B. Indications for intubation/tracheal suctioning

V. **Care of the Neonate with Possible Diaphragmatic Hernia**

Chapter 18 Questions
Neonatal Resuscitation

1. Which of the following statements regarding secondary apnea of the newborn is TRUE?
   a. It is immediately preceded by a rise in heart rate and blood pressure.
   b. Adequate tactile and thermal stimulation or very brief artificial ventilation during this period will trigger respiratory effort.
   c. During this period, the newborn shuts down peripheral circulation so that color changes from blue to white.
   d. It is possible with thorough examination of tone, breathing effort, color, and heart rate, to know whether a newborn is in secondary rather than primary apnea at birth.

2. Which of the following is NOT an effect of hypoxia in the newborn?
   a. Persistent fetal circulation
   b. Build up of carbon dioxide
   c. Vasodilation of the pulmonary vasculature
   d. Metabolic acidosis

3. Of the following situations leading to the need for resuscitation, which is the MOST common?
   a. Birth trauma
   b. Fetal asphyxia
   c. Maternal medication
   d. Fetal malformations

4. Which of the following steps in newborn resuscitation should always be undertaken FIRST?
   a. Assess respirations
   b. Evaluate heart rate
   c. Clear the airway
   d. Evaluate color

◼ **DATA FOR ITEM 5**

A newborn under your care has no spontaneous respiratory effort. Tactile stimulation and clearing of the airway does not stimulate spontaneous respirations.

5. What is the MOST appropriate step to take next in the resuscitation of this newborn?
   a. Evaluate heart rate
   b. Provide 100% free-flow oxygen
   c. Perform immediate endotracheal intubation
   d. Provide positive-pressure ventilation with 100% oxygen

◼ **DATA FOR ITEM 6**

You have been providing positive pressure ventilation with 100% oxygen to a newborn under your care. After 30 seconds you check the newborn's heart rate and find that it is 88 bpm and not increasing.

6. What is the MOST appropriate step to take next in the resuscitation of this newborn?
   a. Discontinue positive-pressure ventilation and provide 100% free-flow oxygen
   b. Continue positive-pressure ventilation for another 30 seconds and then reevaluate the heart rate
   c. Continue positive-pressure ventilation and begin chest compressions for 30 seconds and then reevaluate the heart rate
   d. Initiate medications to increase the heart rate

DATA FOR ITEM 7

You have been providing ventilation in combination with chest compressions to a newborn under your care for 60 seconds. When you recheck the infant's heart rate, you find that it is 68 bpm and not increasing.

7. **What is the MOST appropriate step to take next in the resuscitation of this newborn?**
   a. Discontinue positive-pressure ventilation and provide 100% free-flow oxygen
   b. Continue positive-pressure ventilation for another 30 seconds and then reevaluate the heart rate
   c. Continue positive-pressure ventilation and chest compressions for 30 seconds and then reevaluate the heart rate
   d. Initiate medications to increase the heart rate

8. **What is the pressure needed for the first newborn breath?**
   a. 10 to 20 cm H_2O
   b. 20 to 30 cm H_2O
   c. 30 to 40 cm H_2O
   d. 40 to 50 cm H_2O

9. **At what rate should breaths be delivered with positive-pressure ventilation (PPV) during resuscitation of the newborn?**
   a. 20 to 40 breaths per minute
   b. 40 to 60 breaths per minute
   c. 60 to 80 breaths per minute
   d. 80 to 100 breaths per minute

10. **Which of the following is NOT an indication for endotracheal intubation of the newborn?**
    a. When a diaphragmatic hernia is suspected
    b. When the newborn needs prolonged ventilation
    c. When adequate oxygenation cannot be achieved with a bag and mask
    d. When you need to alleviate gastric/abdominal distention

DATA FOR ITEM 11

You are listening to a newborn's chest to check to see if there was adequate placement of the endotracheal tube. You hear breath sounds on both sides of the chest, but they sound louder on the right side. There does not appear to be a rise and fall of the chest as air moves in and out.

11. **Based on these findings, you suspect that the endotracheal tube is MOST likely placed in which of the following positions?**
    a. The esophagus
    b. In the mid-tracheal region
    c. In the larynx
    d. In one of the main bronchus

DATA FOR ITEM 12

You are conducting resuscitation efforts on a newborn, who despite positive pressure ventilation and chest compressions, has a heart rate of 62 beats per minute. You decide to administer some epinephrine.

12. **What is the correct dose of 1:10,000 concentration epinephrine to administer to a neonate?**
    a. 0.1 to 0.3 mL/kg
    b. 0.4 to 0.6 mL/kg
    c. 1 to 3 mL/kg
    d. 4 to 6 mL/kg

13. Which of the following statements regarding care of the neonate born in meconium-stained fluid is TRUE?

    a. For all infants who have passed meconium in utero, a through suctioning of the head as it rests on the perineum and before the body is born is indicated.

    b. When suctioning meconium-stained fluid, you should always suction the nose before you suction the mouth and pharynx.

    c. A DeLee suction trap is the ideal method for achieving safe and thorough suctioning of the newborn.

    d. In order to perform adequate deep suctioning of the trachea, a suction tube should be passed through the endotracheal tube.

14. Which of the following statements about the use of Apgar scores during neonatal resuscitation is TRUE?

    a. The Apgar score can predict whether there has been any permanent brain damage due to the asphyxia.

    b. The Apgar score can be used to determine whether a newborn needs resuscitation at birth.

    c. The Apgar score can be used to evaluate whether resuscitation efforts have been successful.

    d. The Apgar score can be used to determine when to stop resuscitation efforts on the newborn.

Chapter 18 Answer Key
Neonatal Resuscitation

1. *c* p. 570

2. *c* p. 570

3. *b* p. 573

4. *c* p. 574

5. *d* p. 574

6. *b* p. 574

7. *d* p. 574

8. *d* p. 575

9. *b* p. 576

10. *d* p. 577

11. *d* p. 578

12. *a* p. 579

13. *a* p. 580

14. *c* p. 571

Chapter 19 Outline
Newborn Examination

I.   Risk Assessment/Chart Review

    A. Environmental/Genetic factors

    B. Social factors

    C. Maternal medical factors

    D. Prenatal factors

    E. Neonatal factors

II.   Gestational Age Assessment

    A. The New Ballard Scale (NBS)

        1. Neuromuscular maturity

            a. Posture

            b. Square window

            c. Arm recoil

            d. Popliteal angle

            e. Scarf sign

            f. Heel to ear

        2. Physical maturity

            a. Skin

            b. Lanugo

            c. Plantar surface

            d. Breast

            e. Eye/Ear

            f. Genitals

        3. Maturity rating

    B. Birthweight and Gestational Age

        1. Small for gestational age (SGA)

        2. Average/Appropriate for gestational age (AGA)

        3. Large for gestational age (LGA)

III.   Anthropomorphic Measurements

    A. Weight

    B. Length

    C. Head circumference

    D. Chest circumference

IV.   Examination

Know Assessment Technique, Parameters of Normal, Variations of Normal, Deviations from Normal, and Assessment for Birth Defects and Genetic Disease.

A. General Appearance
   1. Color Assessment
      a. Cyanosis/Acrocyanosis
      b. Ecchymosis
      c. Mongolian spots
      d. Jaundice
   2. Posture
   3. Tone
   4. Alertness and Cry

B. Cardiopulmonary System Assessment
   1. Respiratory effort
   2. Respiratory rate
   3. Thorax excursion
   4. Anteroposterior chest diameter
   5. Breath sounds
   6. Heart rate/rhythm
   7. Heart sounds
   8. Apical pulses

C. Skin Assessment
   1. Moisture
   2. Temperature
   3. Peeling
   4. Vernix
   5. Lanugo
   6. Milia
   7. Erythema toxicum
   8. Mottling

D. Head Assessment
   1. Head circumference/Head to body ratio
   2. Head shape
   3. Molding
   4. Sutures
   5. Fontanelles
   6. Caput succedaneum
   7. Cephalohematoma
   8. Head lag
   9. Hair distribution

E. Facial Assessment
   1. Positioning/relation of eyes, ears, nose, mouth

F. Oral Assessment
  1. Mouth
     a. Position
     b. Shape and size
  2. Mucous membranes
  3. Chin
  4. Lips
  5. Palate
  6. Tongue
  7. Uvula
  8. Gag reflex
  9. Sucking reflex
  10. Rooting reflex
  11. Salivation

G. Nose Assessment
  1. Position
  2. Nares
  3. Olfactory response

H. Eyes Assessment
  1. Position
  2. Shape and size
  3. Sclera
  4. Conjunctiva
  5. Iris
  6. Pupils
  7. Cornea
  8. Retina
  9. Visual response
  10. Lacrimal duct
  11. Blink reflex
  12. Red reflex
  13. Doll's-eye reflex

I. Ears Assessment
  1. Position
  2. Shape and size
  3. Skin tags
  4. Cartilage formation
  5. Auditory response
  6. Otoscopic examination

J. Neck Assessment
  1. Shape
  2. Length
  3. Tonic neck reflex
  4. Thyroid
  5. Lymph nodes

6. Carotid pulse

7. Clavicles

K. Abdomen and Thorax Assessment

  1. Chest circumference

  2. Chest/thoracic tympany

  3. Diaphragm excursion

  4. Ribs

  5. Xyphoid process

  6. Breast

  7. Areola

  8. Shape of abdomen

  9. Umbilical cord

 10. Abdominal musculature

 11. Bowel sounds

 12. Abdominal palpation

    a. Kidneys

    b. Liver

    c. Spleen

    d. Bladder

    e. Femoral pulse

    f. Hernias

 13. Abdominal tympany

L. Genitourinary Tract Assessment (Female)

  1. Labia majora

  2. Labia minora

  3. Clitoris

  4. Urethral meatus

  5. Vagina

  6. Perineum

  7. Anus

  8. Anal wink

M. Genitourinary Tract Assessment (Male)

  1. Penis

  2. Urinary meatus

  3. Urinary stream

  4. Testes and scrotum

  5. Perineum

  6. Anus

  7. Anal wink

N. Upper Extremities Assessment

  1. Length

  2. Range of motion

    a. Shoulder

    b. Clavicles

    c. Elbow

    3. Wrist

       a. Square window

    4. Hand

       a. Grasp reflex

    5. Scarf sign

    6. Arm recoil

    7. Palm

    8. Fingers

    9. Nails

   10. Clavicles

   11. Pulses

O. Lower Extremities Assessment

    1. Length

    2. Toes

    3. Feet

    4. Ankle dorsiflexion

    5. Popliteal angle

    6. Heel-to-ear maneuver

    7. Nails

    8. Plantar creases

    9. Buttocks

   10. Range of motion

   11. Hips

       a. Ortolani's maneuver

       b. Barlow's maneuver

   12. Knee jerk/patellar reflex

   13. Plantar reflex

P. Back

    1. Spinal column

    2. Vertebrae

Q. Neurological Examination

    1. Response to stimulation

    2. Assessment of senses

       a. Optic

       b. Olfactory

       c. Auditory

    3. Assessment of Reflexes

       a. Face/Mouth

          i. Rooting reflex

         ii. Sucking reflex

        iii. Gag reflex

       b. Eyes

          i. Pupillary reflex

         ii. Red reflex

        iii. Doll's eye reflex

        iv. Blink reflex

  c. Upper extremities

    i. Palmar grasp reflex

  d. Lower extremities

    i. Patellar reflex

    ii. Plantar reflex

    iii. Step reflex

    iv. Babinski reflex

  e. Torso

    i. Anal wink

    ii. Tonic neck reflex

  f. Moro reflex

Chapter 19 Questions
Newborn Examination

1. What is the minimum gestational age for which the New Ballard Scale (NBS) is accurate?
   a. 20 weeks
   b. 24 weeks
   c. 26 weeks
   d. 28 weeks

2. What is the margin of error for the New Ballard Scale (NBS)?
   a. 1 week
   b. 2 weeks
   c. 3 weeks
   d. 4 weeks

■ **DATA FOR ITEM 3**

With the infant supine and the pelvis flat on the examining surface, the leg is flexed on the thigh at the knee and the thigh is fully flexed using one hand; the leg is then extended at the knee while keeping the thigh flexed.

3. These are the instructions to conduct which of the following neuromuscular maturity evaluations?
   a. Square window
   b. Leg recoil
   c. Popliteal angle
   d. Heel to ear

4. Which of the following is an anthropomorphic measurement of the newborn?
   a. Square window angle
   b. Degree of arm recoil
   c. Birth weight
   d. Popliteal angle

5. The presence of how many minor malformations is suggestive of a major underlying malformation in the newborn?
   a. 2
   b. 3
   c. 4
   d. 5

6. Which of the following is the MOST commonly used criteria for the evaluation of the neurological status of the newborn?
   a. The rooting reflex
   b. The palmar grasp reflex
   c. The Moro reflex
   d. The Babinski reflex

7. Persistence of the entire Moro reflex beyond what age following a term birth is considered ABNORMAL?
   a. 1 month
   b. 2 months
   c. 3 months
   d. 4 months

8. Which of the following is TRUE regarding the presence of vernix?
   a. It increases with gestational age
   b. It decreases with gestational age
   c. It is unrelated to gestational age

9. A high-pitched cry is indicative of which of the following abnormalities?
   a. Seizures
   b. Increased intracranial pressure
   c. Prematurity
   d. Respiratory distress

10. Which of the following findings upon inspection of the skin of the newborn is NOT an indicator of prematurity?
   a. Absence of vernix
   b. Abundance of lanugo
   c. Visible veins across the abdomen
   d. Mottling

11. As you are examining the head of a newborn you note that there is an area of swelling of the scalp that extends over the suture lines. Which of the following BEST describes this finding?
   a. Overriding sutures
   b. Molding
   c. Caput succedaneum
   d. Cephalohematoma

12. As you are examining a term newborn, her mother asks when the "soft spot" on the baby's head will disappear. Which of the following is the best answer to this question?
   a. Within the first month of life
   b. Within the first six months of life
   c. At approximately 12 to 18 months of life
   d. At approximately 24 months of life

13. Which of the following findings upon examination of a newborn's eyes would be considered ABNORMAL?
   a. Red eye reflex
   b. Doll's-eye response
   c. Blink response
   d. Sunset eyes

14. What is the normal range for head circumference for the average full-term newborn?
   a. 28 to 32 centimeters
   b. 32 to 38 centimeters
   c. 38 to 42 centimeters
   d. 42 to 46 centimeters

15. A positive result on the Ortolani or Barlow maneuvers signals to which of the following neonatal abnormalities?
   a. Prematurity
   b. Neurological damage or immaturity
   c. Congenital hip dysplasia
   d. Osteogenesis imperfecta

■ DATA FOR ITEM 16

As you are examining a newborn shortly after birth you note the following:

Arms are fully flexed at elbows while legs are extended

You can flex the wrist completely against the forearm without effort

There is almost no lanugo present, the body is mostly bald

Creases are present over 2/3 of the anterior portion of the sole of the foot

There is some cracking of the skin and a few veins are visible

The ear pinna are well formed and firm, there is instant recoil

16. These findings indicate that the newborn is MOST likely which of the following gestational ages?

    a. 35 weeks

    b. 37 weeks

    c. 40 weeks

    d. 42 weeks

Chapter 19 Answer Key
Newborn Examination

1. *a* p. 586

2. *b* p. 586

3. *c* p. 587

4. *c* p. 589

5. *b* p. 590

6. *c* p. 592

7. *d* p. 592

8. *a* p. 870

9. *b* p. 871

10. *d* p. 872–873

11. *c* p. 873–874

12. *c* p. 874

13. *d* p. 877

14. *b* p. 873

15. *c* p. 885

16. *c* p. 587

Chapter 20 Outline
The Sick Newborn

I. **Respiratory Dysfunction**

   A. Signs/Symptoms of respiratory distress

   B. Transient tachypnea of the newborn (TTN)

   C. Respiratory distress syndrome (RDS)/Hyaline membrane disease

   D. Pneumothorax

   E. Pneumonia

   F. Persistent pulmonary hypertension of the newborn

   G. Meconium aspiration syndrome

   H. Apnea

   I. Diaphragmatic hernia

   J. Congenital heart disease

   K. Choanal atresia

   Know the following for each of the above conditions:
      1. Signs/Symptoms
      2. Etiology
      3. Immediate/Supportive management and care

II. **Cardiovascular Dysfunction**

   A. Murmurs

   B. Congenital heart defects

   Know the following for each of the above conditions:
      1. Signs/Symptoms
      2. Etiology
      3. Immediate/Supportive management and care

III. **Gastrointestinal Dysfunction**

   A. Cleft palate/Cleft lip

   B. Esophageal atresia/Esophageal fistula

   C. Omphalocele/Gastroschisis

   D. Necrotizing enterocolitis

Know the following for each of the above conditions:
1. Signs/Symptoms
2. Etiology
3. Immediate/Supportive management and care

IV. Metabolic Dysfunction

A. Hypoglycemia

B. Hypergylcemia

C. Hypocalcemia

Know the following for each of the above conditions:
1. Signs/Symptoms
2. Etiology
3. Immediate/Supportive management and care

V. Infections

A. Signs/Symptoms of infection

B. Bacterial infections
1. Group Beta Streptococcus (GBS)
2. E. coli

C. Viral infections

Know the following for each of the above conditions:
1. Signs/Symptoms
2. Etiology
3. Immediate/Supportive management and care

VI. Birth Injuries

A. Cephalohematoma/Skull fractures

B. Facial palsy/Brachial plexus injuries

C. Bone fractures

Know the following for each of the above conditions:
1. Signs/Symptoms
2. Etiology
3. Immediate/Supportive management and care

VII. Central Nervous Disorders and Neurological Dysfunction

A. Seizures

B. Meningocele

C. Meningomyelocele

Know the following for each of the above conditions:
1. Signs/Symptoms
2. Etiology
3. Immediate/Supportive management and care

VIII.   Drug Exposure

A. Signs/Symptoms

B. Immediate/Supportive management and care

IX.   Growth Disorders

A. Macrosomia

B. Intrauterine growth retardation (IUGR)

Know the following for each of the above conditions:

1. Signs/Symptoms

2. Etiology

3. Immediate/Supportive management and care

Chapter 20 Questions

The Sick Newborn

■ **DATA FOR ITEM 1**

You are examining a newborn 6 hours after birth. The infant is cyanotic and there appears to be some chest distension over the left side. On auscultation you note that there are diminished breath sounds over the left lung field.

1. Based on these findings, which of the following conditions would you MOST suspect?
   a. Tracheal-esophageal fistula
   b. Pneumothorax
   c. Neonatal pneumonia
   d. Transient tachypnea of the newborn

2. Which of the following mechanisms is responsible for transient tachypnea of the newborn?
   a. Air from the lungs is pushed outward from the alveoli into an atypical space
   b. Meconium particles in the lungs that lead to air trapping, hypoxia, air leaks, and persistent pulmonary hypertension
   c. Inadequate absorption of liquid from the lungs after birth
   d. Inadequate levels of surfactant to maintain patency of the alveoli

3. Which of the following is the MOST common sign of neurological compromise in the newborn period?
   a. A high-pitched cry
   b. Spasticity of the limbs
   c. Seizure activity
   d. Increased irritability and jitteriness

■ **DATA FOR ITEM 4**

A newborn under your care is born with eviscerated abdominal organs that are covered by a membranous sac.

4. Which of the following terms is used to describe this condition?
   a. Gastroschisis
   b. Omphalocele
   c. Meningocele
   d. Meningomyelocele

5. In addition to a STAT call to the pediatric team, what is the midwifery management of a diaphragmatic hernia diagnosed at birth?
   a. Positive pressure ventilation with a bag and mask
   b. Immediate endotracheal intubation and artificial ventilation
   c. Administration of epinephrine at the recommended dose for newborns
   d. Immediate chest compressions and positive pressure ventilation with bag and mask

A newborn in your care develops severe respiratory distress immediately after birth. You note decreased breath sounds in the left lung field, heart sounds predominantly on the right side of the chest, and a concave abdominal contour.

6. Based on these findings, you would MOST suspect which of the following conditions?
   a. Esophageal atresia
   b. Ventral septal defect
   c. Tracheal-esophageal fistula
   d. Diaphragmatic hernia

7. Midwifery management of esophageal atresia includes positioning of the newborn in which of the following positions?
   a. Prone
   b. Supine
   c. Left-lateral
   d. Right-lateral

8. Neonatal abstinence syndrome is MOST associated with which of the following drug exposures of the fetus in utero?
   a. Tobacco
   b. Cocaine
   c. Heroin
   d. Alcohol

9. Which of the following is the MOST appropriate management of a neonate whom you suspect has been drug-exposed in utero?
   a. Talk to the mother and see if she will admit any drug use to you
   b. Report your suspicions to child welfare officials
   c. Report your suspicions to the police
   d. Order a urine toxicology screen on both the newborn and the mother

10. The infant of a diabetic mother is at increased risk for all of the following EXCEPT:
   a. Early jaundice
   b. Tremors
   c. Hyperglycemia
   d. Polycythemia

The parents of an infant who is suffering from Erb-Duchenne paralysis ask you about the prognosis for their infant.

11. Your answer to their questions should be based on which of the following?
   a. Knowledge that the majority of these cases of paralysis disappear in 3 to 6 months
   b. Knowledge that this type of paralysis often leads to respiratory compromise due to paralysis of the phrenic nerve, which innervates the diaphragm
   c. Knowledge that this type of paralysis usually requires corrective surgery and physical therapy at approximately 6 months of age
   d. Knowledge that this paralysis is temporary and will likely disappear within the first month of life

12. Which of the following scenarios is MOST likely to result in brachial plexus injury?
   a. Forceps delivery that leads to bruising of the facial nerve
   b. Breech delivery in which traction was applied to the neck
   c. Abnormal fetal position which lead to prolonged pressure on the fetal face from the maternal sacrum
   d. Delivery of an arm in a compound presentation by sweeping the arm across the chest and over the head

13. Which of the following is the MOST appropriate management step to take when you suspect that a newborn has a congenital viral or bacterial infection?

    a. Order that blood, throat, and urine cultures be taken directly from the newborn

    b. Order that the cord blood be saved for testing or culture

    c. Perform a heel stick on the newborn to send for culture

    d. Wait until the pediatric team is contacted before taking any action

14. Which of the following should be the TOP priority in the midwife's management plan for the care of a newborn who appears to have an early-onset bacterial infection?

    a. Coordinating/ensuring adequate respiratory support efforts

    b. Contacting the pediatric team

    c. Initiating antibiotic treatment

    d. Obtaining the necessary lab work such as blood cultures and chest X-ray

15. What is the most common type of seizure activity in the newborn?

    a. Multi-focal

    b. Focal

    c. Tonic-clonic

    d. Subtle

DATA FOR ITEM 16

A newborn under your care exhibits the following:

Birthweight of 5 lb. 12 oz.

Head circumference 28 centimeters

Loose skin around the shoulders and back

Dry, peeling skin that is meconium stained

Prominent eyes

16. Based on these findings you MOST suspect which of the following?

    a. Fetal alcohol syndrome

    b. Postmaturity syndrome

    c. Intrauterine growth retardation (IUGR)

    d. Prematurity

DATA FOR ITEM 17

During a home visit to a woman at 10 days postpartum you note that the newborn seems lethargic. The mother states that she has had an increasingly difficult time feeding the infant and that he seems to sleep more than her other children did when they were infants. Upon examination of the baby you note that his skin has a slight grayish color to it. His heart rate is 178 beats per minute and his respirations are 70 breaths per minute.

17. Based on these findings you MOST suspect which of the following?

    a. Neonatal abstinence syndrome

    b. Failure-to-thrive

    c. Congenital heart disease

    d. Transient tachypnea of the newborn

Chapter 20 Answer Key
The Sick Newborn

1. *b* p. 610

2. *c* p. 611

3. *c* p. 613

4. *b* p. 613

5. *b* p. 614

6. *d* p. 614

7. *a* p. 614

8. *c* p. 615

9. *d* p. 615

10. *c* p. 616

11. *a* p. 612–613

12. *b* p. 612

13. *b* p. 611

14. *a* p. 611

15. *d* p. 613

16. *c* p. 616

17. *c* p. 612

Chapter 21 Outline
Primary Care of the Newborn

For this entire section, know how to explain/teach to the parents the following infant-care basics.

I.   Newborn Behavior

    A. Sleep-Wake States

        1. Brazelton's Categorization of Infant Behavioral States

    B. Newborn reflexes

    C. Sensory capabilities

    D. Regulation of behavior

    E. Developmental milestones

    F. Psychological tasks

II. Infant Growth/Weight Gain

    A. Parameters of Normal

    B. Management of abnormal growth/weight gain

III. Maternal-Infant Bonding

    A. Parameters of Normal

    B. Assessment/Facilitation of maternal-infant bonding

    C. Management of abnormal bonding process

IV. Newborn Screening Tests

    A. Hearing tests

    B. Phenylketonuria (PKU)

    C. Galactosemia

    D. Homocystinuria

    E. Hypothyroidism

    F. Maple syrup urine disease

    G. Sickle cell anemia

    Know the following for each of the above tests:

        1. Definition/Description of condition being tested for

        2. Management of abnormal test results

V.   Infant/Childhood Immunizations

    A. Immunization schedule

    B. Signs/symptoms of allergic reaction to immunization

VI. Baths/Skin Care

A. Technique

B. Safety consideration

VII. Umbilical Cord Care

A. Cleaning technique

B. Signs/symptoms of abnormal umbilical cord healing

VIII. The Circumcision Decision

A. Pro's and con's of circumcision

B. Contraindications to circumcision

IX. Circumcision Care

A. Cleaning technique

B. Signs/Symptoms of abnormal circumcision site healing

X. Non-nutritive sucking

A. Definition

B. Decision to use pacifier

XI. Feeding

A. Breastfeeding (This topic is also discussed in Chapter 22)
   1. Frequency
   2. Technique

B. Formula feeding
   1. Frequency
   2. Amount
   3. Technique
   4. Choice of formula
   5. Cow milk allergies/Lactose intolerance

C. Vitamin/Mineral supplementation

D. Eating patterns

E. Weight gain

F. Introduction of solids

XII. Diaper Rash

A. Irritative diaper dermatitis

B. Signs/Symptoms

C. Etiology/Predisposing factors

D. Management/Treatment

E. Monilial diaper rash

F. Signs/Symptoms

G. Etiology/Predisposing factors

H. Management/Treatment

XIII. Cradle Cap

A. Signs/symptoms

B. Etiology

C. Management

XIV. Mouth Thrush

A. Signs/Symptoms

B. Etiology

C. Management

XV. Fussy Baby/Colic

A. Management

B. Coping strategies

XVI. Jaundice

A. Physiological vs. pathological jaundice

B. Management of pathologic jaundice

XVII. Safety Considerations

A. Car seats

B. Reducing risk of SIDS

C. Pets

Chapter 21 Questions
Primary Care of the Newborn

■ **DATA FOR ITEM 1**

TM is a new mother in to see you for an appointment at 2 weeks postpartum. The prenatal course and birth were normal and the infant is healthy. The woman is concerned because her mother has been telling her that it is unhealthy for the baby to be picked up every time she cries. She wants to know your opinion on dealing with a crying newborn.

1. Which of the following would be the MOST appropriate response to TM's concerns?
   a. To tell her that her mother is right—a newborn needs to learn self-soothing behavior and that this will only happen if it is allowed to cry itself to sleep
   b. To tell her that once she has checked to make sure that her baby does not need to be fed or changed, she should put the infant down and that eventually she will fall asleep on her own
   c. To tell her that newborns usually only cry when they need to be fed or changed or when they are in pain, so that crying should always be investigated for one of these causes
   d. To explain to her that newborns have a primal need to be held and that crying is often an expression of this need, which needs to be met and which will not lead to spoiling

2. Approximately what percentage of a normal newborn's time is spent sleeping?
   a. 40%
   b. 50%
   c. 60%
   d. 70%

3. The American Academy of Pediatrics Task Force on Infant Positioning and Sudden Infant Death Syndrome (SIDS) recommends which of the following positions for sleeping newborns?
   a. Supine
   b. Prone
   c. Lateral
   d. Semi-recumbent

4. What is the rate of complications from circumcision of the male newborn?
   a. 1%
   b. 2 to 5%
   c. 10%
   d. 15%

5. Which of the following BEST describes the method for cleaning the penis of the newborn while a circumcision is healing?
   a. Gently wiping with a gauze covered with Vaseline or A & D ointment
   b. Using lukewarm water only
   c. Using lukewarm water and a mild, hypoallergenic soap
   d. Applying alcohol with cotton swabs to the base of the circumcision

6. When can parents begin to give their babies tub baths rather than sponge baths?
   a. Approximately one week after birth
   b. When the circumcision and umbilical sites have healed
   c. When the infant has enough tone in its neck muscles to hold its head up
   d. When the infant can sit up in the tub with minimum support

7. What is the minimum age at which an infant can start drinking cow's milk?
   a. 3 months
   b. 6 months
   c. 12 months
   d. 24 months

8. At what age do formula-fed infants need to start receiving iron supplementation?
   a. 2 months
   b. 3 months
   c. 4 to 6 months
   d. 6 to 8 months

9. What mineral other than iron needs to be supplemented in a breastfed infant?
   a. Calcium
   b. Zinc
   c. Copper
   d. Fluoride

10. For a normal term newborn what is the caloric requirement for formula?
   a. 20 cal/oz
   b. 24 cal/oz
   c. 26 cal/oz
   d. 28 cal/oz

11. Approximately how much breastmilk/formula should a term infant receive at each feeding during the first two weeks of life?
   a. 10 to 20 mL
   b. 30 to 60 mL
   c. 70 to 90 mL
   d. 100 to 120 mL

12. Which of the following statements about weight gain in infants is FALSE?
   a. During the first few days of life (3 to 5 days), healthy term newborns may lose 5 to 10 percent of their birthweight.
   b. Over the course of the first year of life, the birthweight of a healthy term newborn quadruples.
   c. Healthy term newborns can be expected to gain approximately 1 ounce per day in weight.
   d. Breastfed newborns usually experience a larger weight loss following birth than formula-fed newborns.

13. Which of the following findings would suggest pathological jaundice instead of physiological jaundice?
   a. Jaundice peaks at day 3 to 4 of life
   b. Jaundice is visible within the first 24 hours of life
   c. Lab tests reveal a predominance of unconjugated bilirubin
   d. Jaundice is not visible after 10 days

14. How often does an infant usually need to eat during the first month of life?
   a. Every 1 to 2 hours
   b. Every 2 to 3 hours
   c. Every 4 to 5 hours
   d. Every 5 to 6 hours

15. Which of the following is a reason for physiological rather than pathological jaundice?
   a. Isoimmunity
   b. Polycythemia
   c. Decreased life span of red blood cells
   d. Pyloric stenosis

16. Which of the following vaccinations for infants and children should NOT be given prior to 12 months of age?

    a. Hepatitis B virus vaccine (HBV)

    b. Diptheria toxoid, tetanus toxoid, whole-cell pertussis vaccine (DTP)

    c. Oral poliovirus vaccine (OPV)

    d. Measles, mumps, and rubella vaccine (MMR)

17. In which of the following waking behavioral states of the newborn, as defined by Brazelton, does the newborn learn best?

    a. Crying

    b. Considerable motor activity

    c. Alert

    d. Drowsy

DATA FOR ITEMS 18–19

You are examining a newborn at 6 weeks of age. You note that it has a rash in the diaper area with erythematous confluent lesions, marked skin-fold involvement, and "satellite" lesions on the abdomen, thighs, and lower back. The infant appears to be in pain as a result of the rash.

18. Based on these findings you MOST suspect which of the following conditions?

    a. Irritative diaper dermatitis

    b. Monilial diaper rash

    c. Beginnings of a varicella rash

    d. Pytyriasis rosea

19. Which of the following is the BEST treatment for this type of rash?

    a. Gentle cleansing with mild soap and tepid water and leaving the area uncovered whenever possible

    b. Zinc oxide barrier cream such as Desitin

    c. Topical nystatin or miconozole

    d. Oral antifungal treatment

Chapter 21 Answer Key
Primary Care of the Newborn

1. *d* p. 596–597

2. *c* p. 597

3. *a* p. 601

4. *a* p. 897

5. *b* p. 897

6. *b* p. 897–898

7. *c* p. 602

8. *b* p. 602

9. *d* p. 602

10. *a* p. 602

11. *b* p. 604

12. *b* p. 607

13. *b* p. 607

14. *b* p. 607

15. *c* p. 869

16. *d* p. 597

17. *c* p. 596, 598

18. *b* p. 605

19. *c* p. 605

PART VI: POSTPARTUM CARE

PART VI

Chapter 22 Outline
The Normal Peurperium

I.   Definition of the Peurperium

II.   Uterine Involution
 A. Definition
 B. Parameters of normal
 C. Assessment

III.   Lochia
 A. Definition
 B. Parameters of normal
 C. Assessment

IV.   Postpartum Changes of Other Organs
 A. Vagina and Perineum
  1. REEDA scale for healing of perineum
 B. Breasts
  1. Anatomy and physiology of lactating breast
  2. Onset of lactation
   a. Milk production
   b. Secretion/Let-down
  3. Maintenance of lactation
 C. Vital signs
 D. Renal system
 E. Weight loss
 F. Hematological changes

V.   Normal Psychological Processes of the Peurperium
 A. Early parental attachment and bonding
 B. Postpartal and early caretaking period
 C. Postpartum/Baby blues
 D. Grief Process/Psychological response to loss
 Know the following for each of the above processes:
  1. Parameters of normal
  2. Facilitation of normal psychological processes
  3. Management of abnormalities

VI.   Management of the Early Peurperium

A. Perineal care

B. Breast care

C. Diet and ambulation

D. Contraception plan

E. Laboratory screening for complications

F. Rh immune globulin (RhoGAM)

G. Rubella immunization

VII.   Postpartal Discomforts

A. After-birth pains/cramping

B. Excessive perspiration

C. Breast engorgement

D. Perineal pain

E. Constipation

F. Hemorrhoids

Know the following for each of the above discomforts:

   1. Etiology
   2. Parameters of normal
   3. Relief measures

VIII.   Breastfeeding

A. Proper positioning

B. Proper latch-on

C. Feeding patterns/frequency

D. Breast care

E. Management of breastfeeding problems

   1. Sore/bleeding/cracked nipples
   2. Inverted or flat nipples
   3. Infant latch-on difficulties
   4. Milk volume/Infant weight gain
   5. Pumping
   6. Engorgement
   7. Mastitits
   8. Candidiasis

F. Maternal medications and lactation

IX. Anticipatory Guidance

A. Perineal care

B. Breast care

C. Abdominal tightening exercises

D. Kegel exercises

E. Activity/Exercise

F. Nutrition

G. Rest

H. Hygiene

I. Baby blues vs. Postpartum depression

J. Maternal warning signs/symptoms/When to call

K. Contraception

L. Sexual intercourse

M. Infant feeding

N. Circumcision care

O. Cord care

P. Infant bathing/Skin care

Q. Holding/Carrying/Comforting infant

R. Stool and urination frequency

S. Diapers/Diapering

T. Diaper rash

U. Taking infant's temperature

V. Well-child visits/Pediatrician choice

W. Infant warning signs/symptoms/When to call

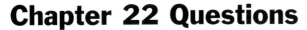
Chapter 22 Questions

The Normal Puerperium

1. Which of the following BEST defines the postpartal period?
  a. From delivery of the placenta to the return of the woman's reproductive tract to its prepregnant condition
  b. From delivery of the placenta to the return of the woman's reproductive tract to its nonpregnant condition
  c. From delivery of the placenta to approximately 6 weeks afterwards
  d. From delivery of the placenta to approximately 8 weeks afterwards

2. How long does the normal puerperium usually last?
  a. 4 weeks
  b. 6 weeks
  c. 8 weeks
  d. 10 weeks

3. By what time after birth is the regeneration of the endometrium completed at all sites except the placental site?
  a. 1 week
  b. 10 days
  c. 2 weeks
  d. 3 weeks

4. By what week after birth has the uterus returned to its nonpregnant weight?
  a. 2 weeks
  b. 4 weeks
  c. 6 weeks
  d. 8 weeks

5. Which of the following findings would be abnormal on the 14th day postpartum?
  a. Uterine fundus palpable at 2 to 3 finger-breadths above the symphysis pubis
  b. Lochia alba
  c. Diastasis recti
  d. Absence of vaginal rugae

6. Which of the following BEST describes the trigger that causes lactogenesis (milk production) during the first 3 to 4 postpartum days?
  a. Fall in progesterone and estrogen levels
  b. Increase in human placental lactogen (HPL)
  c. Suckling by the newborn
  d. Supression of oxytocin release

7. Which of the following hormones is predominantly responsible for milk ejection?
  a. Human placental lactogen (HPL)
  b. Progesterone
  c. Prolactin
  d. Oxytocin

8. Which of the following statements concerning milk production and milk ejection is FALSE?

   a. For women who do not breastfeed, milk production will occur but milk secretion will not take place.

   b. Fear and anxiety can prevent milk ejection in a breastfeeding woman.

   c. Let-down and ejection of milk can be triggered in a breastfeeding woman without the actual suckling of the infant.

   d. Once lactation is successfully initiated, milk production will continue even without suckling stimulation on the breast.

9. Which of the following findings would be ABNORMAL in a woman in the early postpartal hours?

   a. Fundus palpable at or above the level of the umbilicus

   b. Significantly increased urine output

   c. Pulse rate of 50 beats per minute

   d. Temperature of 101°F

10. Rh immune globulin (RhoGAM) should be administered postpartally to which of the following?

   a. An infant with Rh positive blood born to a mother with Rh negative blood with a positive direct-Coomb's test

   b. A woman with Rh negative blood with an infant with Rh positive blood with a negative direct-Coomb's test

   c. A woman with Rh negative blood with an infant with Rh negative blood with a negative direct-Coomb's test

11. Which of the following statements regarding breast engorgement is TRUE?

   a. Bromocriptime (Parlodel) is the preferred medication to treat engorgement in non-breastfeeding women.

   b. It lasts approximately 3 to 4 days.

   c. It is an inflammatory process that often causes a low-grade fever.

   d. It is caused by milk and lymphatic stasis.

12. Which of the following is an appropriate measure to relieve breast engorgement in a non-breastfeeding woman?

   a. Manually express milk to relieve pressure

   b. Apply warmth to the breasts

   c. Bromocriptine to suppress lactation

   d. Apply a breast binder

◼ DATA FOR ITEM 13

A woman in the third post-partum day is having sharp nipple pain while breastfeeding and her nipples are cracked.

13. Which of the following is the MOST likely cause of this problem?

   a. Lack of proper nipple care following each feeding

   b. An infant with a vigorous suckling pattern

   c. Improper positioning of the infant at the breast

   d. Failing to break the suction before removing the baby from the breast

14. How soon after a vaginal birth can a woman begin doing Kegel and chin-chest tucks for abdominal tightening?

   a. 1–2 days

   b. 1 week

   c. 2 weeks

   d. 4 weeks

Chapter 22 Answer Key
The Normal Peurperium

1. *b* p. 623

2. *b* p. 623

3. *d* p. 623

4. *d* p. 624

5. *a* p. 624

6. *a* p. 625–626

7. *d* p. 626

8. *d* p. 626

9. *d* p. 627, 526

10. *c* p. 639–640

11. *d* p. 643–644

12. *d* p. 644–645

13. *c* p. 650

14. *a* p. 652–653

Chapter 23 Outline
Complications of the Puerperium

I. Puerperal Morbidity

    A. Definition

        1. Puerperal morbidity vs. puerperal infection

    B. Differential diagnosis

        1. Dehydration

        2. Urinary tract infections (UTI's)

        3. Upper respiratory tract infections (URI's)

        4. Mastitis

        5. Puerperal infections

    C. Management/Treatment

II. Puerperal Infection

    A. Definition

    B. Predisposing causes

    C. Etiology

        1. Infection resulting from trauma to vulva, perineum, vagina, or cervix

        2. Endometritis

        3. Pelvic cellulitis (Parametritis)

        4. Peritonitis

        5. Septic thrombophlebitis

        6. Bacteremia

    D. Signs/Symptoms

    E. Management/Treatment

III. Mastitis/Breast Abscess

    A. Definition

    B. Etiology

    C. Signs/Symptoms

    D. Management/Treatment

IV. Thrombophlebitis/Pulmonary Embolism

    A. Definition

    B. Etiology

    C. Signs/Symptoms

    D. Management/Treatment

V.   Hematomas

    A. Definition

    B. Etiology

    C. Signs/Symptoms

    D. Management/Treatment

VI.   Late Postpartum Hemorrhage

    A. Definition

    B. Etiology

    C. Signs/Symptoms

    D. Management/Treatment

VII.   Subinvolution

    A. Definition

    B. Etiology

    C. Signs/Symptoms

    D. Management/Treatment

        1. Methylergovine (Methergine) series

VIII.   Postpartum Depression

    A. Definition

    B. Etiology

    C. Predisposing causes

    D. Signs/Symptoms

        1. Postpartum/Baby blues vs. Postpartum depression

    E. Management/Treatment

IX.   Failure to Thrive

    A. Definition

    B. Etiology

    C. Predisposing causes

    D. Signs/Symptoms

    E. Management/Treatment

X.   Child Abuse/Maternal Rejection

    A. Definition

    B. Etiology

    C. Predisposing causes

    D. Signs/Symptoms

    E. Management/Treatment

Chapter 23 Questions
Complications of the Puerperium

1. Which of the following women would be considered to be suffering from puerperal morbidity as defined by the Joint Committee on Maternal Welfare?
   a. A woman who is 20 hours postpartum and whose last two temperatures were 100.8°F and 101.2°F
   b. A woman who is in the fourth day postpartum and who today has a temperature of 101.0°F
   c. A woman who is in the ninth day postpartum and who yesterday had a temperature of 100.6°F and today has a temperature of 101.4°F
   d. A woman who is the second postpartum day (38 hours postpartum) whose last two temperatures were 100.2°F and 101.6°F and who yesterday had temperature of 101.2°F

2. Which of the following conditions would be considered a puerperal infection?
   a. Urinary tract infection
   b. Septic thrombophlebitis
   c. Mastitis
   d. Upper respiratory infection

■ **DATA FOR ITEM 3**

You are evaluating FJ, a 32-year-old G3P2112 in the fourth postpartum day who over the last 36 hours has had a fever ranging from 100.88 to 103.08F. She had an uncomplicated prenatal course with twins with the exception of two urinary tract infections that were successfully treated. Her intrapartum course was complicated by a third degree laceration and an immediate postpartum hemorrhage for which bimanual uterine compression was applied. Below are your findings on physical exam:

Blood pressure: 130/78

Temperature: 102.68F

Heart rate: 110 beats per minute

Lungs: Clear bilaterally to auscultation

Breasts: Tender, slightly engorged bilaterally, cracked nipples

Abdomen: Fundal height 1 fingerbreadth below umbilicus; lower abdominal and uterine tenderness on palpation, negative costovertebral angle tenderness (CVAT); slight abdominal distension

Lochia: Scant, odorless

Perineum: 38 laceration repair, edges well approximated, moderately edematous

Extremities: Within normal limits with the exception of +1 pedal edema

3. Given your findings from her chart and your physical exam, which of the following is the MOST likely cause of FJ's symptoms?
   a. Urinary tract infection/pyelonephritis
   b. Peritonitis
   c. Endometritis
   d. Mastitis

4. Which of the following is the advice to give a breastfeeding woman with mastitis regarding continuation of breastfeeding?

   a. That she will need to discontinue breastfeeding for the duration of the necessary antibiotic treatment, but that she can resume breastfeeding after the infection is cleared

   b. That she will need to discontinue breastfeeding in order to allow the tissue to heal and the infection to resolve

   c. That she should continue to breastfeed and should increase the frequency of feedings to prevent stasis

   d. That she should continue to breastfeed on the unaffected breast and either manually express or pump the affected breast to promote healing

DATA FOR ITEM 5

A woman in the second postpartum day is complaining of pain in her left leg. Upon examination you note that she has a slight temperature (99.4°F), a pulse of 86, and that an area on her left calf is warm to touch, extremely tender, and red.

5. Which of the following is MOST likely to cause these symptoms?

   a. Inflamed varicose veins

   b. Superficial venous thrombophlebitis

   c. Deep vein thrombophlebitis

   d. Septic thrombophlebitis

6. Which of the following is contraindicated in the management of thrombophlebitis?

   a. Elevation of the affected extremity

   b. Hot packs applied to the affected extremity

   c. Therapeutic massage to the affected extremity

   d. Elastic stockings

7. In addition to postpartum "blues" and postpartum psychosis, what other conditions should be included in your differential diagnosis list for postpartum depression?

   a. Sheehan's syndrome

   b. Asherman's syndrome

   c. Postpartum thyroiditis

   d. Hashimoto's disease

8. Which of the following is the treatment of choice for uterine subinvolution diagnosed at a 4-week postpartum visit?

   a. Uterine exploration/dilation and curettage (D & C)

   b. Ibuprofen (Motrin) and uterine massage

   c. Broad-spectrum antibiotics

   d. Methylorgonovine (Methergine)

Chapter 23 Answer Key
Complications of the Peurperium

1. *c* p. 673

2. *b* p. 674

3. *c* p. 675

4. *c* p. 678

5. *b* p. 678

6. *c* p. 678

7. *c* p. 680

8. *d* p. 680

PART VII

PRACTICE TESTS

Chapter 24
Practice Test 1

■ **DATA FOR ITEM 1**

"Nurse-midwives believe that every individual has a right to safe, satisfying health care with respect for human dignity and cultural variations."

1. The quote above is the opening sentence to which of the following ACNM documents?
   a. The Code of Ethics
   b. The Definition of Nurse-Midwifery Practice
   c. The Standards for the Practice of Nurse-Midwifery
   d. The Philosophy of the American College of Nurse-Midwifery

■ **DATA FOR ITEM 2**

As you examine a woman's vagina and perineum during the fourth stage of labor, you notice that she has a laceration that involves the vaginal mucosa, posterior fourchette, perineal skin, perineal muscles, and the external anal sphincter.

2. This laceration is classified as which of the following?
   a. A first degree laceration
   b. A second degree laceration
   c. A third degree laceration
   d. A fourth degree laceration

3. What is the normal range for chest circumference for the average full-term newborn?
   a. 30 to 36 centimeters
   b. 36 to 42 centimeters
   c. 42 to 48 centimeters
   d. 48 to 52 centimeters

4. Which of the following women is MOST likely to suffer from mastitis?
   a. A breastfeeding woman in the first 7 days postpartum
   b. A breastfeeding woman more than a week postpartum
   c. A non-breastfeeding woman in the first 7 days postpartum
   d. A non-breastfeeding woman more than a week postpartum

■ **DATA FOR ITEMS 5–6**

BN, a 33-year-old G4P1111 at 26 weeks gestational age, was in a motor vehicle accident (MVA) in which she sustained significant blood loss. She is in stable condition now. Her laboratory results reveal the following: Hemoglobin 9 ml/dL; elevated reticulocyte count; and a mean corpuscular volume of 86.

5. These results suggest which of the following?
   a. Macrocytic anemia
   b. Microcytic anemia
   c. Normocytic anemia
   d. Hemolytic anemia

6. Which of the following is the MOST appropriate treatment for BN's anemia at this time?
   a. Folic acid supplementation
   b. Iron supplementation
   c. Packed red blood cell transfusion
   d. Vitamin B12 supplementation

DATA FOR ITEM 7

During an abdominal examination of a woman at term you feel the cephalic prominence on the same side as the fetal parts.

7. This is indicative of which of the following?
   a. Face presentation
   b. Vertex (occipital) presentation
   c. Brow presentation
   d. Sinciput (military) presentation

8. Early decelerations of the fetal heart rate are thought to be caused by which of the following?
   a. Impending birth
   b. Head compression
   c. Uteroplacental insufficiency
   d. Cord compression

9. Which of the following pharmacological agent is MOST effective in the treatment of bacterial vaginosis?
   a. Metronidazole p.o.
   b. Metronidazole vaginal gel
   c. Clindamycin p.o.
   d. Amoxicillin p.o.

10. Which of the following BEST describes the role of the midwife following an abnormal result on a genetic screening test?
   a. To help the woman and her partner cope with the results and help them to prepare for their child's special needs.
   b. To transfer care of the woman to a physician who specializes in high-risk pregnancies.
   c. To explain and schedule appropriate follow-up diagnostic tests.
   d. To transfer care to a genetic counselor who can best serve the needs of the couple.

DATA FOR ITEM 11

A pelvic exam on a woman with vaginal spotting and abdominal pain reveals that the woman's cervix is long and closed, that she has tenderness on right side especially with movement of the cervix, and that there is a small mass in the right adenexal area. She does not have a fever, has some nausea but no vomiting, and her last menstrual period was approximately five weeks ago.

11. Which of the following do you MOST suspect?
   a. Appendicitis
   b. Salpingitis
   c. Impending abortion
   d. Ectopic pregnancy

12. If engagement took place in LOT position, how many degrees does the fetal head rotate during internal rotation for an occiput-anterior delivery?
   a. 45
   b. 90
   c. 135
   d. 180

13. Approximately how many times should a healthy, well-hydrated infant void during a 24 hour time period?

  a. 3 times

  b. 4 times

  c. 5 times

  d. 6 times

■   DATA FOR ITEM 14

The following are the findings of clinical pelvimetry performed on DS, a 30-year-old G1P0:

Inlet – anterior, lateral, and posterior segments are well rounded; transverse diameter about the same as the anteroposterior diameter

Sacrum – parallel with the symphysis pubis

Sacrosciatic notch – well rounded

Sidewalls – straight

Ischial spines – blunt, non-encroaching, not prominent

Pubic arch – approximately 90 degrees

14. Based on this information, which of the following BEST describes DS's type of pelvis?

  a. Android

  b. Anthropoid

  c. Gynecoid

  d. Platylpelloid

15. A wandering baseline is associated with which of the following?

  a. Administration of drugs such as butorphanol (Stadol) and meperidine (Demerol)

  b. Impending fetal demise

  c. Rapid descent of the fetal head

  d. Maternal fever/infection

16. How soon after a full-term delivery can a woman who is not breastfeeding safely start taking combination oral contraceptives?

  a. Immediately

  b. 1 week

  c. 3 weeks

  d. 6 weeks

■   DATA FOR ITEM 17

DA comes to your office complaining of painful and "itchy" bumps on her vagina. Upon examination you note a half-dozen vesicles on her labia minora and majora. DA states that she has had a fever and general malaise for about 5 days. She has some inguinal lymphadenopathy.

17. Which of the following is the MOST likely cause of these findings?

  a. Secondary syphilis

  b. Herpes simplex virus

  c. Human papillomavirus

  d. Bartholin's cysts

18. When is maternal to infant (vertical) transmission of the human immunodeficiency virus (HIV) MOST likely to happen?
   a. In the first 20 weeks of pregnancy
   b. In the third trimester
   c. During labor and delivery
   d. During breastfeeding

19. If a woman is Rh-negative and unsensitized, approximately when in pregnancy should she receive Rh immune globulin (RhoGAM) to prevent possible Rh sensitization?
   a. 20 weeks
   b. 28 weeks
   c. 32 weeks
   d. 36 weeks

■ **DATA FOR ITEM 20**

A prenatal client at 30 weeks gestation has an abnormal fasting blood glucose and an abnormal 1-hour glucose challenge test.

20. What is the MOST appropriate action at this time?
   a. Order a repeat 1-hour glucose challenge test
   b. Rescreen at 34–36 weeks gestation
   c. Diagnose this client as a gestational diabetic and consult with a physician
   d. Order a 3-hour glucose tolerance test (GTT)

21. Which of the following describes the normal uterine contraction pattern?
   a. Contraction of equal strength but different durations throughout the uterus
   b. Contraction of longer and stronger duration in the fundus to minimal or nonexistent toward the cervix
   c. Contraction of longer and stronger duration in the cervix to minimal or nonexistent toward the fundus
   d. Contraction of equal strength and equal duration at the fundus and cervix

22. The anterior fontanel is roughly the shape of:
   a. A rhomboid
   b. A diamond
   c. A triangle
   d. An oval

23. What is the most common cause of uterine rupture?
   a. Separation of a previous cesarean section scar
   b. Congenital anomalies of the uterus
   c. Labor stimulation/augmentation with oxytocin or prostaglandins
   d. External cephalic version

24. Which of the following findings would be considered ABNORMAL in a newborn at approximately 90 minutes following birth?
   a. A state of deep, unresponsive sleep
   b. A light murmur audible on auscultation
   c. Absence of bowel sounds
   d. A heart rate of 108 bpm

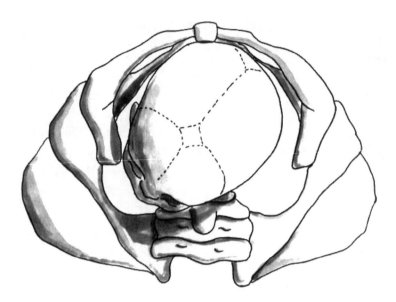

25. The drawing above illustrates which of the following?
   a. A fetal head in LOA position
   b. A fetal head in ROA position
   c. A fetal head in ROP position
   d. A fetal head in LOP position

26. Which of the following BEST describes the trigger that causes milk ejection from the breast?
   a. Fall in progesterone and estrogen levels
   b. Increase in human placental lactogen (HPL)
   c. Suckling by the newborn
   d. Supression of oxytocin release

■   **DATA FOR ITEM 27**

A newborn under your care is exhibiting symptoms of hypoglycemia so you decide to perform a heel stick on the infant to determine his glucose level. The results reveal that this infant's glucose level is 42 mg/dL.

27. What is the MOST appropriate action to take at this time?
   a. Attempt to get the newborn to feed and repeat the glucose test in 30 minutes
   b. Note in the chart that the glucose level is within normal limits for a newborn within 24 hours of birth
   c. Attempt to get the newborn to feed and place the newborn under a radiant warmer
   d. Notify the pediatrician/pediatric team so that they can order intravenous fluids containing glucose

28. Which of the following baseline fetal heart rates is considered the cut-off for marked bradycardia?
   a. Below 110 beats per minute
   b. Below 100 beats per minute
   c. Below 90 beats per minute
   d. Below 80 beats per minute

■ **DATA FOR ITEM 29**

CT had a positive urine pregnancy test today in your office. She states that she had a period on 4/2/00 that lasted the normal length of 5 days with heavy flow on the first 2 days and lighter bleeding for the rest of the period. On 4/29/00 she had another menstrual period of approximately the same duration and quantity. On 5/19/00 she had her period once again, but it was shorter, lasting 2 to 3 days, and lighter than usual in quantity of flow. Today she presents with some spotting that has been going on for 2 days.

29. In order to estimate CT's gestational age by LMP you would use which date?
   a. 4/2/00
   b. 4/29/00
   c. 5/19/00

■ **DATA FOR ITEM 30**

JC is a client who uses combination oral contraceptives and has been having breakthrough bleeding between periods for 6 months. JC continues to have breakthrough bleeding despite previous measures to try to solve this problem. She has regular menstrual periods/withdrawal bleeding during her week of placebo pills and her history reveals that she has been taking her pills correctly.

30. What is the MOST appropriate action to take at this time?
   a. Recommend that she use a back-up method until the bleeding has stopped, and reassure her that in most cases breakthrough bleeding will remit on its own
   b. Have her come in to your office so that you can perform an exam and rule out pregnancy
   c. Have her come in to your office so that you can switch her to another pill or start her on a new contraceptive method
   d. Have her come in to your office so that you can switch her to a non-hormonal method of contraception

31. The biophysical profile score for a 36-year-old G5P2123 at 40 weeks gestational age by ultrasound is of 6/10 with an abnormal AFV. Which of the following is the MOST appropriate management plan?
   a. Reassess BPP within 24 hours
   b. Admit to hospital and maintain under constant observation
   c. Give the mother corticosteroids and assess fetal lung maturity in 24 hours
   d. Recommend immediate delivery for fetal indications

32. Which of the following changes in cervical mucus signals the "peak day" in the menstrual cycle during which ovulation is most likely to occur?
   a. The first day during which the cervical mucus is thick, sticky, and tacky
   b. The first day in which the cervical mucus is clear, slippery, and stretchy
   c. The last day during which the cervical mucus is thick, sticky, and tacky
   d. The last day during which the cervical mucus is clear, slippery, and stretchy

33. At which of the following times is maternal cardiac output highest?
   a. Before 20 weeks of pregnancy
   b. After 20 weeks of pregnancy
   c. During labor
   d. Immediately postpartum

34. How is fetal station determined?

   a. By measuring the distance of the widest diameter of the fetal presenting part above or below the ischial spines

   b. By measuring the distance of the lowermost part of the fetal presenting part above or below the ischial spines

   c. By measuring the distance of the widest diameter of the fetal presenting part above or below the pelvic inlet

   d. By measuring the distance of the lowermost part of the fetal presenting part above or below the pelvic inlet

35. Which of the following describes the accurate infiltration site for a pudendal block?

   a. Immediately anterior to the ischial spine as it passes the anterior surface of the sacrospinous ligament and into Alcock's canal

   b. Immediately anterior to the ischial spine but posterior to the sacrospinous ligament

   c. Immediately posterior to the ischial spine and through the sacrospinous ligament

   d. Immediately posterior to the ischial spine and anterior to the sacrospinous ligament

DATA FOR ITEM 36

CK is a 28-year-old G3P2002 at approximately 32 weeks gestational age. Today she is measuring size-greater-than-dates. You note that she has some generalized edema, especially of the lower extremities. You have difficulty palpating fetal position and auscultation fetal heart tones.

36. Based on this information, you MOST suspect which of the following?

   a. Multiple gestation

   b. Preeclampsia

   c. Polyhydramnios

   d. Macrosomia

37. Which of the following would be part of your work-up to confirm your diagnosis?

   a. PIH labs

   b. Amniocentesis

   c. Non-stress test

   d. Ultrasound

38. Which of the following is NOT an indication for artificial rupture of membranes during first stage of labor?

   a. To speed up a normal labor

   b. To attach an internal fetal monitor

   c. To facilitate the descent of the fetal head

   d. To reduce the possibility of a sudden and vigorous spontaneous rupture of membranes

DATA FOR ITEM 38

Twenty minutes after delivery of an infant, the placenta has not delivered. You have attempted draining the placenta, putting the baby to breast, and emptying the woman's bladder via catheterization. The nurse informs you that the woman has developed tachycardia and when you touch the woman she feels cold and clammy. She complains that she feels weak and "weird." You perform another vaginal exam to see if the placenta has moved into the lower uterine segment or vaginal vault. You feel a soft, tumor-like projection filling the cervical opening and with your abdominal hand you feel a funnel-like depression instead of the uterine fundus.

39. These findings are MOST suggestive of which of the following third stage complications?

    a. Placenta accreta

    b. Placental separation with occult hemorrhage

    c. Uterine inversion

    d. Endometritis

■ **DATA FOR ITEM 39**

    You are conducting an exam on a newborn at 3 weeks of life while he is quiet and alert. You note that despite repeated efforts, you cannot elicit either a Moro or a grasping reflex from the infant. Both these reflexes were present in the newborn at birth.

40. What is the MOST appropriate response to this finding?

    a. Note it as a normal finding in a quiet and alert behavioral state

    b. Note it as a normal finding in an infant of this age that is beginning to develop increased neurological maturity

    c. Note it as a variation from normal that in absence of any other neurological variations will not need additional medical attention

    d. Note it as an alarming variation from normal that merits immediate attention by a pediatrician

41. Which of the following is TRUE of chloasma?

    a. It is the increased pigmentation of the aerola and of the midline of the abdomen (linea nigra).

    b. It occurs only during pregnancy.

    c. It is most noticeable in brunettes.

    d. It is considered a precursor to melanoma.

42. If a fetus suffers from malnutrition during the time of development when cells are increasing in number, then the damage suffered by the fetus is BEST characterized as which of the following?

    a. Irreversible

    b. Reversible

    c. Asymmetric

    d. Catabolic

■ **DATA FOR ITEM 42**

    On vaginal exam of a breech presentation you feel the sacrum in the left, transverse portion of the maternal pelvis.

43. Which of the following is used to describe this fetus' variety and position?

    a. LOT

    b. LST

    c. Frank LOT

    d. Frank LST

44. If engagement occurred in the LOP position and birth occurred in the OP position, external rotation will bring the fetal head into which of the following positions?

    a. LOA

    b. LOT

    c. LOP

    d. OP

45. Which of the following findings on the examination of a term newborn at 76 hours following birth would be considered ABNORMAL?

    a. Cyanosis of the hands and feet

    b. Slight ecchymosis over the presenting part

    c. Mongolian spots on the buttocks

    d. Facial jaundice

46. Which of the following statements indicates that a woman has understood how to properly use a female condom?
    a. "Both the flexible rings must be placed inside the vagina, one against the cervix past the pubic bone and one right inside the vagina in front of the pubic bone."
    b. "To remove the female condom, I should reach in and pull on the rim of the ring that is sitting against the cervix, just like removing a diaphragm."
    c. "I should not leave the condom in for more than six hours."
    d. "To remove the female condom, I should squeeze and twist the outer ring and then pull out the condom using the outer ring."

■ **DATA FOR ITEM 46**

When you come out of the hospital room of one of your clients you notice that there is a man in scrubs and with a hospital ID that is looking through your client's medical chart. You do not recognize this person as a member of the Obstetrical and Gynecological service at the hospital. When you approach him he states that he is your client's brother and that he is also a resident within the Orthopedics service at the hospital. His hospital ID confirms this information.

47. Which of the following describes the BEST management of this situation?
    a. Since he is a physician within the hospital, you allow him to continue reading your client's chart.
    b. You find one of the residents from the Obstetrics and Gynecology service and ask her to resolve the situation.
    c. You tell him that since he is the client's brother he should not be reading the chart although he is a physician in the hospital and would otherwise be allowed to read this chart.
    d. You remind him that client's charts are confidential regardless of the fact that he is a physician in the hospital and that he needs his sister's explicit consent before reading the chart.

■ **DATA FOR ITEM 47**

LK, a 36-year-old G2P0010, presents with vaginal bleeding at 35 weeks gestation. She complains of colicky uterine pain. Upon abdominal examination you feel mild, discoordinate contractions. The uterus is indentable during the contractions and the uterus is neither board-like nor rigid between contractions, but she does have pain with palpation. The fetal heart rate is 120 with repeated late decelerations.

48. Based on LK's symptoms you MOST suspect which of the following?
    a. Placenta previa
    b. Placental abruption
    c. Uterine rupture
    d. Premature labor

■ **DATA FOR ITEM 48**

As the placenta is expelled, you notice that the fetal side of the placenta is presenting.

49. Which of the following statements is true about this type of placental presentation?
    a. It is called the Schultz mechanism and results from placental separation that begins centrally.
    b. It is called the Duncan mechanism and results from placental separation that begins centrally.
    c. It is called the Schultz mechanism and results from separation that begins at the margin or periphery of the placenta.
    d. It is called the Duncan mechanism and results from a separation that begins at the margin or periphery of the placenta.

50. Which of the following is NOT a potential complication of maternal human papillomavirus (HPV) infection during pregnancy?
   a. Increase in number and size of warts
   b. Excessive bleeding during delivery if tearing or cutting extends to affected region
   c. Intrauterine infection of fetus with the virus
   d. Intrapartum laryngeal infection of neonate

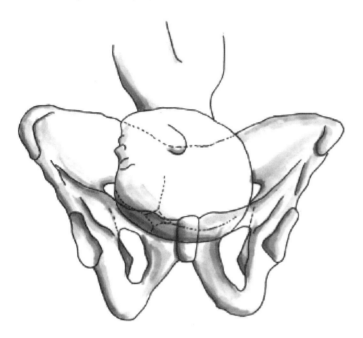

51. The drawing above BEST illustrates which of the following?
   a. A fetus in LOT position with anterior asynclitism
   b. A fetus in LOT position with posterior asynclitism
   c. A fetus in ROT position with anterior asynclitism
   d. A fetus in ROT position with posterior asynclitism

52. For which of the following patients is watchful waiting NOT appropriate when there is painless vaginal bleeding in the first trimester?
   a. A woman with three previous SAB's
   b. A woman with previous tubal surgery
   c. A woman who is pregnant with twins
   d. A woman who you suspect has a blighted ovum

53. Birth of the head occurs through which of the following mechanisms for an occiput-posterior delivery?
   a. Flexion
   b. Extension
   c. Flexion then extension
   d. Extension then flexion

54. Where is the uterine fundus normally palpated in the immediate postpartum period (after delivery of the placenta)?
   a. At the level of the umbilicus
   b. Approximately two-thirds of the way between the symphysis pubis and the umbilicus
   c. Approximately 1–2 finger breadths above the umbilicus
   d. Approximately 1–2 finger breadths above the symphysis pubis

55. A newborn with a gastroschisis is MOST at risk for which of the following complications?
    a. Hyperthermia
    b. Seizures
    c. Hypoglycemia
    d. Dehydration

56. Which of the following BEST describes Norplant's main mechanism of action?
    a. Modification of fallopian tube motility, which affects speed of ovum transport
    b. Supression of ovulation by complete suppression of follicle-stimulating hormone (FSH) and luteinizing hormone (LH)
    c. Creation of an atrophic endometrium that is hostile to implantation by a fertilized ovum
    d. Thickening of the cervical mucus, which prevents passage of sperm

57. According to the American College of Obstetricians and Gynecologists (ACOG), what score on the Bishop Pelvic Scoring system is favorable and likely to result in a successful labor induction?
    a. A score of at least 4
    b. A score of at least 6
    c. A score of at least 8
    d. A score of at least 10

■ **DATA FOR ITEM 57**

HG is a 29-year-old G2P2002 who is in to see you because she has been having heavy and prolonged mid-cycle bleeding with some cramping and pain. She had an IUD inserted 18 months ago and although she had some metrorrhagia for the first 2 months following insertion, she has had no problems since then. Her last menstrual period was normal. You perform a pregnancy test, which is negative. Upon speculum examination you note that strings of her IUD are longer than you noted them on the last examination.

58. Based on this information, which of the following is your MOST likely diagnosis?
    a. Threatened/incomplete abortion
    b. Pelvic inflammatory disease (PID)
    c. Uterine perforation by the IUD
    d. Partial expulsion of the IUD

59. Which of the following is the source of the majority of circulating estrogen in the post-menopausal period?
    a. Conversion of testosterone in the ovary
    b. The primary follicle and corpus luteum in the ovaries
    c. Peripheral conversion of androstenedione in fat cells
    d. Conversion of androstenedione in the adrenal glands

60. The sex of the fetus is clearly distinguishable by direct examination at what gestational age by LMP?
    a. 10th week
    b. 12th week
    c. 14th week
    d. 16th week

61. Using Naegele's rule, what is the estimated due date for a woman whose last menstrual period was 10/25/00?
    a. 08/01/01
    b. 07/31/01
    c. 08/02/01
    d. 07/01/01

62. Which of the following BEST describes the optimal time for folic acid supplementation in order to reduce the risk of neural tube defects?

a. Preconceptually

b. For the first trimester of pregnancy

c. For 1 to 3 months prior to pregnancy and through the first week of pregnancy

d. Prior to conception and through the first six weeks of pregnancy

■ **DATA FOR ITEM 62**

A 24-year-old woman has been exposed to rubella at work. She is currently 27 weeks pregnant. The lab results form her initial prenatal visit indicates that she is rubella non-immune.

63. Which of the following is the MOST appropriate action for you to take next in the management of this client?

a. Watchful waiting to see if she develops clinical signs of disease and if they appear, referral for medical management

b. Administration of hyperimmune gamma globulin if it has been within 96 hours of exposure

c. Order an ultrasound to look for the triad of signs of fetal rubella infection

d. Obtain a blood specimen to test for IgG and IgM antibody titers and consult with a physician

64. Which of the following women should NOT receive a sulfa drug to treat asymptomatic bacteriuria?

a. A woman at 38 weeks gestation

b. A woman at 10 weeks gestation

c. A woman with anemia

d. A woman with sickle cell disease

■ **DATA FOR ITEM 64**

You are performing an abdominal exam on a woman at approximately 16 weeks gestational age.

65. Where would you expect to feel her uterine fundus?

a. Two fingerbreadths above the symphysis pubis

b. Halfway between the symphysis pubis and umbilicus

c. One to two fingerbreadths below the umbilicus

d. At the umbilicus

66. Research supports which of the following approaches to oral intake during labor?

a. Allowing women to drink only water and ice chips during labor

b. Allowing women in normal labor to have clear liquids but no solids during labor

c. Allowing women in normal labor to eat and drink during early stages of labor, but limiting oral intake to liquids as labor progresses

d. Allowing women in normal labor to eat and drink at will throughout the course of their labor

67. According to Friedman, what is the average length of second stage for multiparas?

a. 15 minutes

b. 20 minutes

c. 30 minutes

d. 40 minutes

68. Which of the following is NOT an effect of cold stress on the newborn?

a. Metabolic acidosis

b. Pulmonary vasoconstriction

c. Hypoglycemia

d. Respiratory alkalosis

69. Positive-pressure ventilation of the newborn should continue until which of the following conditions are met?
   a. The heart rate is above 80 beats per minute.
   b. The heart rate is above 100 beats per minute.
   c. There are spontaneous respirations.
   d. There are spontaneous respirations and the infant's color is pink.

70. At what age do breastfed infants need to start receiving iron supplementation?
   a. 2 months
   b. 3 months
   c. 4 to 6 months
   d. 6 to 8 months

Chapter 24 Answer Key

Practice Test 1

1. *d* p. 4
2. *c* p. 865
3. *a* p. 879
4. *b* p. 677
5. *c* p. 346
6. *b* p. 347
7. *b* p. 739
8. *b* p. 478
9. *a* p. 50–51
10. *c* p. 287
11. *d* p. 332
12. *b* p. 437
13. *d* p. 607
14. *c* p. 795
15. *b* p. 481–482
16. *c* p. 120
17. *b* p. 56
18. *c* p. 184
19. *b* p. 357
20. *c* p. 354
21. *b* p. 384
22. *b* p. 401
23. *a* p. 488
24. *c* p. 564

25. *a* p. 398–400
26. *c* p. 626
27. *a* p. 556
28. *b* p. 403
29. *b* p. 255
30. *c* p. 121
31. *d* p. 304
32. *d* p. 75
33. *d* p. 350
34. *b* p. 385
35. *c* p. 818
36. *c* p. 357
37. *b* p. 358
38. *a* p. 419
39. *c* p. 523
40. *d* p. 598
41. *c* p. 230
42. *a* p. 318
43. *b* p. 399
44. *b* p. 440
45. *a* p. 869
46. *d* p. 88
47. *d* p. 348 PM
48. *b* p. 366

49. *a* p. 514
50. *c* p. 58
51. *b* p. 398–401
52. *b* p. 328, 331
53. *c* p. 440
54. *b* p. 525
55. *d* p. 613
56. *d* p. 129
57. *b* p. 473
58. *d* p. 108
59. *c* p. 205
60. *c* p. 241
61. *a* p. 255
62. *d* p. 320
63. *d* p. 340
64. *a* p. 344
65. *b* p. 732
66. *d* p. 410–411
67. *a* p. 433
68. *d* p. 554
69. *c* p. 577
70. *c* p. 602

Chapter 25

Practice Exam 2

■ **DATA FOR ITEM 1**

LK is a 26-year-old nullipara. She is engaged to be married in 3 months and wants a highly effective method of contraception to use instead of condoms, which have been her method of birth control until now. She is interested in a method that has a quick return to fertility because she may desire to become pregnant in 1 or 2 years. Her medical history is unremarkable. Her pelvic exam today reveals a non-parous cervix with no signs of infection and no cervical motion tenderness. Her uterus is markedly retroverted.

1. Which of the following methods of contraception is MOST appropriate for LK?
   a. Diaphragm
   b. Intrauterine device
   c. Depo-Provera
   d. Combination oral contraceptives

2. Which of the following statements describes Piskacek's sign?
   a. It is a sporadic and painless contraction of the uterus that can happen during implantation.
   b. It is an irregularity in the shape of the uterus detectable in the area where the ovum has implanted.
   c. It is a dextro-rotation of the uterus in response to enlargement and increased weight of the fundus.
   d. It is a softening and compressibility of the isthmus of the uterus due to increased vascularity, congestion, and edema.

3. Studies of protein intake among pregnant women in the USA have revealed which of the following?
   a. That usual intake of protein is in excess of the RDA
   b. That usual intake of protein is below the RDA
   c. That usual intake of protein approximates the RDA
   d. That usual intake of protein is not of complete proteins as outlined by the RDA

4. In which days surrounding childbirth is it most likely that maternal varicella infection will be passed to the newborn?
   a. Day 10 before birth to day 5 following birth
   b. Day 2 before birth to day 6 following birth
   c. Day 6 before birth to day 2 following birth
   d. Day 5 before birth to day 10 following birth

5. Which of the following statements is TRUE regarding the accuracy of ultrasound to determine gestational age?
   a. It increases as pregnancy progresses.
   b. It decreases as pregnancy progresses.
   c. The stage of pregnancy does not affect accuracy.
   d. Ultrasound is not an accurate means of determining gestational age.

6. What is the average rate of dilatation during the phase of maximum slope for a multipara?
   a. 1.5 cm per hour
   b. 2.0 cm per hour
   c. 3.2 cm per hour
   d. 5.7 cm per hour

7. Which of the following is the MOST reliable way to detect abnormal or periodic fetal heart rate changes or patterns when using a fetoscope or ultrasound?

   a. Counting the fetal heart rate over the course of 1 minute through a contraction

   b. Counting the fetal heart rate for 15 seconds and multiplying by 4

   c. Counting the fetal heart rate twice for 30 seconds, once during a contraction and once between a contraction

   d. Counting the fetal heart rate in 5-second increments allowing a 5-second break between the period of counting during a contraction

8. Restitution accomplishes which of the following in a birth with cephalic presentation?

   a. Substitutes a larger fetal head diameter for the smaller suboccipitobregmatic diameter

   b. Untwists the fetal neck and brings the head into a right angle with the shoulders

   c. Brings the anteroposterior diameter of the fetal head into alignment with the anteroposterior diameter of the maternal pelvis

   d. Brings the bisacromial diameter of the fetus into alignment with the anteroposterior diameter of the pelvic outlet

9. What is the definition of hypoxemia?

   a. Decreased oxygen in the blood

   b. Decreased oxygen in the tissue

   c. Excessive acidity of the blood

   d. Decreased oxygen in the tissue and metabolic acidosis\

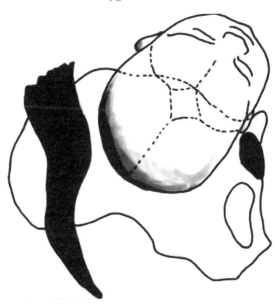

10. The drawing above BEST illustrates which of the following?

   a. Engagement

   b. Anterior asynclitism

   c. Posterior asynclitism

   d. Synclitism

11. Which of the following is MOST directly responsible for closure of the ductus arteriosus?

   a. Decrease in blood pH

   b. Increase in lymph circulation

   c. Increased pressure in the left atrium

   d. Increase in oxygen levels in the blood

12. At what rate should chest compressions be delivered during newborn resuscitation?
    a. 60 compressions per minute
    b. 80 compressions per minute
    c. 90 compressions per minute
    d. 100 compressions per minute

■   **DATA FOR ITEM 13**

The parents of an uncircumcised 12-month-old male infant call you concerned because they cannot retract the foreskin of their infant's penis for routine cleaning.

13. Which of the following responses would be MOST accurate?
    a. The penis probably still has normal adhesions that will work themselves loose with time—usually by the age of 3 years. They should wash the penis without trying to forcefully retract the foreskin.
    b. The penis probably still has normal adhesions that can be worked loose with gentle attempts to retract the foreskin. The adhesions should disappear by 16 months of age.
    c. The infant may be suffering from phimosis—an abnormal inability to retract the foreskin that should be evaluated by a pediatrician or by an urologist.
    d. The infant may be suffering from phimosis—an abnormal inability to retract the foreskin for which a circumcision is indicated.

14. Which of the following is the MOST common cause of uterine subinvolution?
    a. Poor abdominal muscle tone
    b. Retained placental fragments
    c. Myomata
    d. Infection

15. In which of the following decades did the practice of nurse-midwifery enjoy its most rapid and widespread growth?
    a. 1920's
    b. 1940's
    c. 1950's
    d. 1970's

16. What is the reasoning behind having a condom in place before there is any contact between the penis and the female genitalia?
    a. To avoid contact with the pre-ejaculatory fluid, which contains enough sperm to cause pregnancy
    b. To avoid contact with the pre-ejaculatory fluid, which can contain enough pathogens, including HIV, to cause infection
    c. To ensure that the condom is rolled to the base and that there is no leakage of sperm
    d. To allow for the application of adequate lubrication to decrease the chance of the condom tearing

17. Which of the following women is NOT a good candidate for Depo-Provera?
    a. A nulligravida
    b. A woman with liver disease
    c. A woman who desires to become pregnant within the next year
    d. A woman who has seizure disorders

■   **DATA FOR ITEM 18**

A healthy, asymptomatic 60-year-old woman who has decided to initiate hormone replacement therapy in order to reduce her risk of osteoporosis asks you whether she will need to have an endometrial biopsy prior to initiating the hormone therapy.

18. What is your best response to this question?
  a. That an endometrial biopsy is considered routine care for any woman initiating hormone replacement therapy
  b. That since endometrial abnormalities are unusual in asymptomatic women, an endometrial biopsy is not necessary for her before initiating hormone replacement therapy (HRT)
  c. That all women on hormone replacement therapy should have an annual screening endometrial biopsy, so that she will have a biopsy after one year of treatment
  d. That all women on hormone replacement therapy should have an endometrial biopsy every 3 to 5 years but that one is not necessary before initiating the hormone therapy

19. At what point in pregnancy should the maternal serum alphafetoprotein (AFP) or the triple screen be performed?
  a. At 8 to 12 weeks gestational age
  b. At 12 to 15 weeks gestational age
  c. At 15 to 18 weeks gestational age
  d. At 18 to 20 weeks gestational age

20. Which of the following BEST describes the cervix of the average multigravida on the verge of true labor?
  a. 50 to 100 percent effaced with a fingertip to 1 centimeter dilation
  b. 50 to 100 percent effaced with 2 to 3 centimeters dilation
  c. Little or no effacement with a fingertip to 1 centimeter dilation
  d. Little or no effacement with 1 to 2 centimeter of more dilation

21. Which of the following is the largest diameter of the fetal head?
  a. Biparietal
  b. Occipitofrontal
  c. Suboccipitobregmatic
  d. Occipitomental

DATA FOR ITEMS 22–23

FC is the 15-year-old daughter of one of your regular clients. Her mother brought her to see you because she is concerned regarding FC's sexual development. FC has not started to menstruate. On physical exam you note that FC has not started to develop breasts nor does she have any pubic or axillary hair growth.

22. Based on these findings, you MOST suspect which of the following diagnoses?
  a. Primary amenorrhea
  b. Secondary amenorrhea
  c. Dysmenorrhea
  d. Oligomenorrhea

23. Which of the following is the BEST management plan for FC?
  a. Reassess her in one year
  b. Obtain a TSH and prolactin level
  c. Order a progesterone challenge test
  d. Refer her to gynecologist

24. Which of the following terms is used to describe the type of oral hormonal contraception in which the estrogen dosage and type remain constant and the type of progestin remains the same but the level of progestin changes between the first and second week of a 21-day cycle, followed by 7 days of no hormonal intake?
    a. Monophasic
    b. Bipahsic
    c. Triphasic
    d. Minipill

25. When teaching a client about the maternal serum alpha-fetoprotein screening test, it is important to remember that this test has:
    a. A high false-positive rate
    b. Low sensitivity
    c. A high false-negative rate
    d. High specificity

■ **DATA FOR ITEM 26**

KL is a 30-year-old G3P1011 at 12 weeks gestational age by ultrasound performed at 8 weeks. She is here to see you for a routine prenatal appointment. Her pregnancy has been unremarkable thus far with the exception of some vaginal bleeding and lower abdominal pain two weeks ago that resolved spontaneously. Today you cannot locate the fetal heart tones and her uterine size is smaller than dates.

26. You suspect which of the following?
    a. A threatened abortion
    b. An inevitable abortion
    c. An incomplete abortion
    d. A missed abortion

27. Which of the following is the smallest pelvic diameter to which the fetus has to accommodate itself?
    a. The obstetrical conjugate
    b. The conjugata vera
    c. The interspinous diameter
    d. The intertuberous diameter

28. Which of the following findings of fetal heart assessment is MOST ominous?
    a. Persistent fetal tachycardia
    b. Repeated late decelerations
    c. Repeated late decelerations with loss of short-term fetal heart variability
    d. Repeated variable decelerations with "shoulders" (small accelerations right before and after the decelerations)

29. Which of the following vital signs will normally remain elevated in the immediate postpartum and during the fourth stage of labor?
    a. Blood pressure
    b. Pulse
    c. Respirations
    d. Temperature

30. Which of the following is TRUE regarding the presence of lanugo?
    a. It increases with gestational age.
    b. It decreases with gestational age.
    c. It is unrelated to gestational age.

31. Which of the following hormones is predominantly responsible for milk production?
    a. Human placental lactogen (HPL)
    b. Progesterone
    c. Prolactin
    d. Oxytocin

DATA FOR ITEM 32

The Pap smear results of a 28-year-old G1P1001 reveal the presence of a low-grade squamous intraepithelial lesion (LGSIL).

32. What is the BEST management of this client?
    a. Repeat the Pap smear in 3 to 6 months
    b. Repeat the Pap smear in 9 to 12 months
    c. Conduct or refer for colposcopy
    d. Refer to gynecologist/oncologist for biopsy and treatment

33. Which of the following is NOT a hormone synthesized and secreted by the placenta?
    a. Human chorionic gonadotropin (hCG)
    b. Relaxin
    c. Estrogen
    d. Progesterone

DATA FOR ITEM 34

RD, a 26-year-old G2P1001 at 28 weeks estimated gestational age (EGA), comes to see you because she has had high fever, night sweats, and a persistent, productive cough. You note that the Mantoux test (PPD) you performed at her initial prenatal visit was negative.

34. Which of the following is the MOST appropriate action for you to take at this time?
    a. Readminister the purified protein derivative (PPD) to see if she has recently converted
    b. Immunize her with bacillus Calmette-Guerin (BCG) vaccine
    c. Begin empirical treatment with isoniazid (INH)
    d. Order a chest X-ray and sputum culture

35. When diagnosing preeclampsia, which of the following is an accurate definition of hypertension?
    a. A rise of 30 mm of mercury in the systolic pressure and/or rise of 15 mm of mercury in the diastolic pressure over baseline blood pressure
    b. A rise of 20 mm of mercury in the systolic pressure and/or rise of 15 mm of mercury in the diastolic pressure over baseline blood pressure
    c. A rise of 30 mm of mercury in the systolic pressure and/or rise of 10 mm of mercury in the diastolic pressure over baseline blood pressure
    d. A rise of 20 mm of mercury in the systolic pressure and/or rise of 10 mm of mercury in the diastolic pressure over baseline blood pressure

36. Which of the following is a reason to deliver the baby's head between contractions rather than during contractions?
    a. To avoid cord prolapse
    b. To avoid sudden decompression of the fetal chest
    c. To avoid abrupt release of restraining pressure on the head
    d. To avoid fetal heart decelerations

37. What is the most frequent reason for seizures in the neonatal period?
   a. Side effects of maternal medication/drug use
   b. Hypoglycemia
   c. Hyperkalemia
   d. Hypoxic-ischemic encephalopathy

38. How long after birth does complete regeneration of the endometrium at the placental site take?
   a. 1 week
   b. 2 weeks
   c. 4 weeks
   d. 6 weeks

39. Which of the following is the MOST appropriate management of an asymptomatic client who tests reactive on a rapid plasma reagin (RPR) test for syphilis but tests negative on the fluorescent treponomal antibody absorbed (FTA-ABS) test?
   a. Note in the client's chart that she had a past exposure to syphilis, but does not have an active infection at this moment
   b. Commence treatment with Benzathine penicillin
   c. Order a darkfield microscopic examination or other direct examination of exudate
   d. Retest with both RPR and FTA-ABS in 4 to 6 weeks

40. All of the following contribute to the development of hemorrhoids in pregnancy EXCEPT which of the following?
   a. Estrogen-induced relaxation of the large bowel
   b. Progesterone-induced relaxation of the vein walls
   c. Increased pressure of the enlarging uterus causing congestion of pelvic veins
   d. Increased pressure of the enlarging uterus leading to increased venous pressure

41. Which of the following INCREASES absorption of nonheme iron?
   a. Milk
   b. Tea
   c. Meat
   d. Egg whites

DATA FOR ITEM 42

As you perform the first of the Leopold's maneuvers on a woman at 38 weeks gestation, you feel a round and hard fetal part that is readily moveable and ballottable.

42. This is indicative of which of the following?
   a. A breech presentation
   b. A cephalic presentation
   c. An unengaged presenting part
   d. A deflexed attitude

DATA FOR ITEM 43

CV is a 33-year-old G3P1011 at 39 weeks gestation. You admitted her to the hospital three hours earlier at her insistence when she was 50 % effaced, 2 centimeters dilated, and having moderate contractions every 7–10 minutes lasting 20–30 seconds. You have been offering her non-pharmacological pain relief measures but she is repeatedly requesting "something to take the edge off." You perform another vaginal exam and determine that she is now 80% effaced but is still two centimeters dilated. Her contractions are still moderate and every 7–10 minutes but are now lasting 30–45 seconds.

43. Which of the following is the MOST appropriate course of action at this point?
   a. Offer her some Nubain and Vistaril
   b. Rupture her membranes to establish a more effective contraction pattern
   c. Continue with the non-pharmacological pain relief measures
   d. Offer her some Vistaril

44. The problem of shoulder dystocia is fostered if the fetal shoulders attempt to enter the true pelvis with the bisacromial diameter in which of the following pelvic diameters?
   a. Transverse
   b. Oblique
   c. Anteroposterior

DATA FOR ITEM 45

As you perform a check on a woman in the immediate postpartum period you note that her uterus is well contracted, but that she has a steady flow of blood from the vagina. Earlier you performed a thorough evaluation of the placenta and you found it to be complete and intact.

45. What is the MOST appropriate step to take at this time?
   a. Order the administration of an oxytocic agent
   b. Begin bimanual uterine compression
   c. Perform a uterine exploration for placental fragments or cotyledons
   d. Quickly but thoroughly examine the woman for cervical, vaginal, and perineal lacerations

46. Approximately how long should it take for a healthy, term newborn to regain his/her birth-weight?
   a. 3 days
   b. 10 days
   c. 20 days
   d. 30 days

DATA FOR ITEM 47

On speculum and bimanual examination of a woman in to see you for an annual gynecological exam you note that there is some bulging of the anterior vaginal wall that reaches the introitus.

47. How would you BEST classify this finding?
   a. First degree cystocele
   b. Second degree cystocele
   c. First degree uterine prolapse
   d. Second degree uterine prolapse

48. Which of the following substances is associated with a syndrome of fetal anomalies?
   a. Marijuana
   b. Alcohol
   c. Cocaine
   d. Opiates

■ **DATA FOR ITEM 49**

KM is a 24-year-old G4P2102 at 38 weeks gestation with an uncomplicated prenatal course. She calls you at 4:00 p.m. to report that she has not felt her baby move all day.

49. Which of the following should be the FIRST step in your management plan for KM?

a. Take a brief history to see if she truly has been focusing on fetal movement

b. Tell her that she needs to sit and focus on fetal activity for an hour and call you back if she does not feel at least 3 movements in that hour.

c. Have her eat, drink, and rest for one hour and tell her to call you back if in that hour she does not feel the baby move at least three times

d. Have her come to the clinic for an NST

■ **DATA FOR ITEM 50**

You are seeing SD, a 25-year-old G2P0, for her initial prenatal visit at approximately 6 weeks gestational age. She is a swimmer who swims at least an hour daily and competes at swim meets about twice a month. She would like to continue competing only until the end of the current swim season by which time she will be 15 weeks pregnant. She has no medical contraindications to exercise. She wants to know what you recommend.

50. Which of the following is the BEST response?

a. That she should discontinue competition swimming until the end of the first trimester when she is less likely to miscarry

b. That she should discontinue competition swimming, but can continue with her daily work-out as long as she avoids fatigue and overtraining

c. That she can continue competition swimming as long as her maximum heart rate remains below 150 beats per minute, at which point it becomes dangerous for the fetus

d. That she can continue competition swimming as long as she is aware of theoretical concerns and monitors her and her fetus' response to the exercise

51. A woman who is Rh negative has a positive indirect Coomb's test at 28 weeks. What is the MOST appropriate management at this time?

a. Order a direct Coomb's test

b. Administer 300 mcg of Rh immune globulin (RhoGAM)

c. Consult with a physician for management

d. Order a Kleinhauer-Betke test to identify fetal blood cells in maternal circulation

■ **DATA FOR ITEM 52**

A 30-year-old G4P3003 wants to use a diaphragm as her method of contraception. She has never used a diaphragm before. Upon vaginal exam you note that she has poor vaginal tone and a second degree uterine prolapse and that the arch behind her spymphysis pubis is average.

52. Which of the following is the MOST appropriate choice for this woman?

a. A coil spring diaphragm

b. An arcing spring diaphragm

c. A method other than a diaphragm

53. Which of the following statements about starting oral contraceptives is TRUE?

a. Oral contraceptives should only be started on the first day of the menstrual cycle.

b. Oral contraceptives should only be started on the Sunday following the start of the menstrual cycle.

c. Oral contraceptives can be started at any period of the menstrual cycle as long as the woman is not pregnant.

d. Different formulations of oral contraceptives will have different start dates.

54. Which of the following BEST describes the midwife's role in the management of a pregnant client with HIV infection?

  a. The midwife can undertake independent management of this patient's care.

  b. The midwife can undertake independent management of this patient's care unless the CD4 count drops below 200 cell/μI.

  c. The midwife must refer this patient for care to a physician who is an expert in the management of HIV.

  d. The midwife can manage the prenatal care for this patient in collaboration and/or consultation with primary care physician/expert in management of HIV.

55. Which of the following terms is used to describe an increase in the size of existing cells?

  a. Hypertrophy

  b. Hyperplasia

  c. Hypermeiosis

  d. Hypermitosis

56. Which of the following statements about the 1-hour glucose screening test is TRUE?

  a. It has a high rate of false-negatives.

  b. It has a high rate of false-positives.

  c. It can be used alone to diagnose gestational diabetes mellitus (GDM).

  d. It will miss a high percentage of women with abnormal glucose tolerance.

57. When in labor are membranes MOST likely to rupture spontaneously?

  a. During the latent phase

  b. Early in the active phase

  c. At the end of the first stage

  d. Early in second stage

58. The posterior fontanel of the fetal skull is formed by the meeting of which of the following sutures?

  a. Sagittal and coronal

  b. Saggittal, lamboidal, and occipital

  c. Sagittal and lamboidal

  d. Posterior, sagittal, and lamboidal

59. On vaginal exam you feel that the fetus is LOT and that the sagittal suture is midway between the symphysis pubis and the sacral promontory. The head is said to have which of the following?

  a. Anterior asynclitism

  b. Posterior asynclitism

  c. Transverse asynclitism

  d. Synclitism

60. Which of the following describes the technique of progressive relaxation?

  a. Keeping one muscle group relaxed while another muscle group is contracted

  b. Taking a deep breath and letting it out in a heavy sigh after a contraction

  c. Using mental imagery to distract thoughts from painful stimuli

  d. Deliberately tightening a single muscle group as tight as possible and then letting it go as limp as possible and then repeating exercise with different muscle group

61. If engagement took place in LOP position, how many degrees does the fetal head rotate during internal rotation for an occiput-posterior delivery?
   a. 45
   b. 90
   c. 135
   d. 180

62. Which of the following is the MOST accurate definition of prolonged rupture of membranes?
   a. Rupture of membranes more than 12 hours before delivery
   b. Rupture of membranes more than 24 hours before delivery
   c. Rupture of membranes more than 12 hours before onset of labor
   d. Rupture of membranes more than 24 hours before onset of labor

DATA FOR ITEM 63

Electronic fetal heart monitoring of a woman with chronic hypertension in late first stage of labor reveals a prolonged deceleration into the 60's and taking over 90 seconds to return to baseline. This is the second prolonged deceleration in the last 20 minutes.

63. What is the MOST appropriate management of this situation?
   a. Place the woman in Trandelenberg or knee-chest position
   b. Perform an amniofusion
   c. Administer oxygen to the mother at 6–8 L/min and continue to monitor
   d. Call your consulting physician to the room

64. Which of the following describes the Brandt-Andrews maneuver?
   a. Bringing the fingertips of your abdominal hand straight down above the symphysis into the lower abdomen while holding the umbilical cord taut to check for placental separation
   b. Pushing down and toward the umbilicus on the uterus above the symphysis pubis with the palm of your abdominal hand to facilitate placental expulsion after separation
   c. Keeping a hand on the uterine fundus to ascertain shape, position, and consistency of the uterus and prevent premature fundal massage
   d. Exerting pressure on the fundus after placental expulsion to ensure that any clots that may interfere with proper uterine involution are expelled

65. Which of the following placental anomalies would you MOST expect to find in the placenta of a woman with severe chronic hypertension?
   a. Placental tissue that is pale and yellowish-gray
   b. Edema of the placenta
   c. Placental cysts
   d. Extensive infarction of entire cotyledons

66. What gauge suture should you use to repair a tear/incision of the bulbocavernosous muscle?
   a. 2–0
   b. 3–0
   c. 4–0
   d. 5–0

DATA FOR ITEM 67

A newborn under your care exhibits the following at 5 minutes following birth:

Heart rate of 110 bpm

Slow, irregular breathing with grunting and retractions

Some flexion of the extremities

A grimace in response to stimulus

Some cyanosis of the peri-oral area, trunk, and extremities

67. What is the 5-minute Apgar Score for this newborn?
   a. 4
   b. 5
   c. 6
   d. 7

DATA FOR ITEM 68

You have been providing positive pressure ventilation with 100% oxygen to a newborn under your care. After 30 seconds you check the newborn's heart rate and find that it is 62 bpm and not increasing.

68. What is the MOST appropriate step to take next in the resuscitation of this newborn?
   a. Discontinue positive-pressure ventilation and provide 100% free-flow oxygen
   b. Continue positive-pressure ventilation for another 30 seconds and then reevaluate heart rate
   c. Continue positive-pressure ventilation and begin chest compressions for 30 seconds and then reevaluate heart rate
   d. Initiate medications to increase heart rate

DATA FOR ITEM 69

You are examining a newborn 24 hours after birth. You find that her respirations are 72 bpm, that she has intermittent nasal flaring, and that she has rales and rhonci on auscultation. Her temperature is stable and she is not cyanotic.

69. Based on these findings, which of the following conditions would you MOST suspect?
   a. Diaphragmatic hernia
   b. Pneumothorax
   c. Neontal pneumonia
   d. Transient tachypnea of the newborn

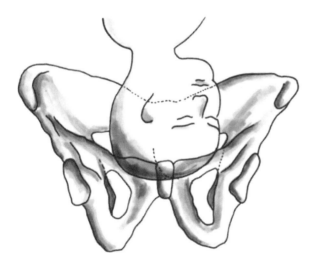

70. The drawing above BEST illustrates which of the following?
   a. A fetal head in LOA position
   b. A fetal head in ROA position
   c. A fetal head in ROP position
   d. A fetal head in LOP position

Chapter 25 Answer Key
Practice Test 2

1. *d*	**25.** *a* p. 285	**49.** *a* p. 293–294
2. *b* p. 234	**26.** *d* p. 329	**50.** *d* p. 144
3. *a* p. 319	**27.** *c* p. 794	**51.** *c* p. 357
4. *c* p. 341	**28.** *c* p. 476–477	**52.** *c* p. 92
5. *b* p. 369–370	**29.** *d* p. 514, 526	**53.** *c* p. 120
6. *d* p. 396	**30.** *b* p. 870	**54.** *d* p. 193
7. *d* p. 404, 417	**31.** *c* p. 625–626	**55.** *a* p. 318
8. *b* p. 437	**32.** *c* p. 46	**56.** *b* p. 353
9. *a* p. 482	**33.** *b* p. 248	**57.** *c* p. 382
10. *b* p. 400–401	**34.** *d* p. 335	**58.** *c* p. 401
11. *d* p. 553	**35.** *c* p. 359–360	**59.** *d* p. 400
12. *c* p. 577	**36.** *c* p. 454	**60.** *d* p. 424
13. *a* p. 601	**37.** *d* p. 613	**61.** *a* p. 440
14. *b* p. 679	**38.** *d* p. 623	**62.** *b* p. 467
15. *d* p. 12	**39.** *d* p. 54	**63.** *d* p. 481
16. *b* p. 86	**40.** *a* p. 269	**64.** *b* p. 516
17. *c* p. 127–128	**41.** *c* p. 320	**65.** *d* p. 836
18. *b* p. 219	**42.** *a* p. 737	**66.** *a* p. 861–862
19. *c* p. 259	**43.** *d* p. 413–415	**67.** *b* p. 562
20. *d* p. 385	**44.** *c* p. 493	**68.** *c* p. 574
21. *d* p. 435	**45.** *d* p. 534	**69.** *d* p. 611
22. *a* p. 60 PM	**46.** *b* p. 607	**70.** *c* p. 398–400
23. *d* p. 60 PM	**47.** *b* p. 768	
24. *b* p. 113	**48.** *b* p. 177	

Notes

Notes

Notes

Notes

Notes

Notes